Chronic Fatigue Syndrome

Chronic Fatigue Syndrome is one of the most enigmatic medical disorders of our time, striking people often in their most productive years. With the controversial debate over cause and treatment of the illness in mind the authors seek to unravel many of the questions surrounding the disorder and its features and characteristics.

Integrating an overview of the latest research with patients' personal experiences and findings, they look at CFS in relation to:

- clinical features
- personal and economic implications
- biological and psychosocial factors
- experiencing symptoms
- coping with the illness.

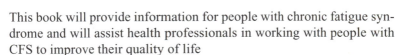

This book will provide information for people with chronic fatigue syndrome and will assist health professionals in working with people with CFS to improve their quality of life

Rona Moss-Morris is a Lecturer and **Keith J. Petrie** is Associate Professor, both at The Faculty of Medical and Health Sciences, The University of Auckland.

The Experience of Illness

Series Editors: Ray Fitzpatrick and Stanton Newman

Other titles in the series

Chronic Fatigue Syndrome

Rona Moss-Morris and
Keith J. Petrie

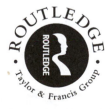

London and New York

NLKIB GWII (F2NY6)

First published 2000
by Routledge
11 New Fetter Lane, London EC4P 4EE

Simultaneously published in the USA and Canada
by Routledge
29 West 35th Street, New York, NY 10001

Routledge is an imprint of the Taylor & Francis Group

© 2000 Rona Moss-Morris and Keith J. Petrie

Typeset in Times New Roman by Bookcraft Ltd, Stroud,
Gloucestershire
Printed and bound in Great Britain by TJ International,
Padstow, Cornwall

British Library Cataloguing in Publication Data
A catalogue record for this book is available from the
British Library

Library of Congress Cataloging in Publication Data
Moss-Morris, Rona, 1962–
   Chronic fatigue syndrome / Rona Moss-Morris and
   Keith J. Petrie.
      p. cm. – (The experience of illness series)
   Includes bibliographical references and index.
   ISBN 0-415-20239-6 – ISBN 0-415-20240-X (pbk.)
   1. Chronic fatigue syndrome.   I. Petrie, Keith J.
   II. Title.   III. Experience of illness.
RB 150.F37 M67 2001
616'.0478—dc21   00-062727

ISBN 0-415-20239-6 (hbk)
ISBN 0-415-20240-X (pbk)

For Grant (RMM) and Cathy (KJP)

Contents

Figures and tables

Figures

Tables

Series editor's preface

Illnesses where the organic basis has yet to be established are always controversial. This is certainly true for chronic fatigue syndrome, which is tackled in this book by Rhona Ross-Morris and Keith Petrie. They deal with the controversy in a systematic fashion, starting off with the historical roots of other diagnoses and conditions that may relate to chronic fatigue syndrome. The nature of the condition involves mental and physical fatigue as well as some pain and muscle weakness, all or some of which most of us have experienced to some degree. The focus of the definition of the illness, as Moss-Morris and Petrie describe, involves a distinct symptom profile and is often used to exclude other psychiatric and medical conditions which may mimic the symptoms of chronic fatigue syndrome. The key area is that of fatigue which has been present for a significant amount of time and does not resolve easily. Although there are differences in the diagnoses used, there has been a development of a new consensus definition which they outline.

The psychological difficulties for patients in dealing with an illness which is not easily attributed to an organic condition, and the different experiences that they have in approaching healthcare professionals, are well described in this book. Petrie and Moss-Morris discuss and analyse the question of whether chronic fatigue syndrome is a unique, specific entity, and how the search for the biological basis of chronic fatigue syndrome has impacted on patients' understanding of the problem that they are experiencing.

The most controversial area concerns the relationship between chronic fatigue syndrome and psychiatric illness. Specifically, chronic fatigue syndrome has been related to anxiety or depression and a disorder where patients have these conditions but relate them to physical complaints. How patients relate their symptoms to a consideration of these having a psychological basis, and the potential stigma associated with a diagnosis of a psychiatric disorder, is well analysed in Chapter 4.

Perhaps the most important issue is that of how patients make sense of their symptoms, and how they think of their condition. Using the illness representations model, Ross-Morris and Petrie carefully analyse the factors that influence patients' representations of chronic fatigue syndrome and how these influence their well-being and behaviour. The most important aspect of this is how patients' cope with their condition. This is outlined in Chapter 7, the final chapter of the volume.

In this volume Ross-Morris and Petrie have made a significant contribution to our understanding of what individuals with chronic fatigue syndrome experience, and how they try to make sense of their symptoms. It will be of interest not only to individuals involved in the treatment of people with chronic fatigue syndrome, but also to individual sufferers themselves. The way in which health care professionals approach the topic, and how this interacts with individuals with chronic fatigue syndrome, will be of particular interest.

Chapter 1

Chronic fatigue syndrome

Then and now

Most of us have felt unduly tired at some time or another. While this sensation is often unpleasant, the impact on our lives is seldom profound. We
may cut down on certain commitments, but in most instances we can continue to perform our day-to-day tasks. However, for some people, like
Judy, the experience of fatigue is devastating and ongoing. In describing
her nine-year battle with fatigue, Judy explains:

> I had no energy or drive whatsoever. I used to feel that I had fifty-
> pound weights on each foot and about thirty-pound weights on each
> wrist. I had this terrible dragging feeling in both the physical and
> mental sense. Writing out a few cheques would be too much. Getting
> the rubbish bags organised and put out on Tuesday mornings was a
> dreaded chore. It was as though I had seized up.
>
> (Judy 1991:39)

Another sufferer of chronic fatigue, Dr Robbie Lopis, a general practitioner, describes how after a viral illness and six weeks rest he returned
to work part time only to find that:

> I could only manage two hours of consulting before I was absolutely
> exhausted. I was forced to move around on a chair with wheels to
> examine patients. I did not have the strength to inflate a baumanometre
> bulb and I had to refer my patients to my partners to have their ears
> syringed as my arms were too weak to draw water into the barrel.
>
> (Lopis 1995:16)

In many cases of profound fatigue a psychiatric or medical diagnosis
can account for these symptoms. However, for some patients, as in Dr

Lopis's case where a 'barrage of medical tests came back normal', such fatigue cannot be explained by any single diagnosis. In these cases fatigue is usually accompanied by a range of other unpleasant symptoms such as mental confusion, muscle and joint pains and severe headaches. Over the past two decades special attention has been given to these patients and the causes of this debilitating fatigue have been hotly debated.

Early reports in the 1980s regarded persistent unexplained fatigue as a psychosomatic reaction to the stressors of modern society. Because the illness appeared largely to afflict young up-and-coming professionals, it became unkindly referred to as 'yuppie flu'. Advocates and sufferers of the illness concurred that the disease was a reaction to the overload of the twentieth century, but strongly rejected the notion that the illness might be psychological in origin (Wessely 1997). Rather, they favoured explanations which included twentieth-century pollutants, toxins, diets, viruses, and weakening of the immune system. A plethora of names for the condition arose, such as chronic immune deficiency syndrome, post-viral fatigue syndrome, and myalgic encephalomyelitis (ME), each reflecting assumptions about the possible organic nature of the illness (Steincamp 1989). In response to the nomenclature controversy and in an attempt to define a homogeneous group of patients for research purposes, the Center for Disease Control and Prevention (CDC) in Atlanta renamed the condition chronic fatigue syndrome or CFS (Holmes *et al.* 1988). Despite claims that CFS is a malady of the past couple of decades, it does in fact have historical predecessors. This chapter reviews the history behind CFS to provide a framework for understanding both the contemporary definitions of the illness and some of the complex sociocultural issues which beset the disorder.

Neurasthenia

Chronic fatigue-like illnesses were described as long ago as the eighteenth century, but the origins of CFS have generally been traced back to the end of the nineteenth century in a condition known as neurasthenia (Shorter 1993; Wessely 1990; White 1989). Neurasthenia was a term coined by an American neurologist, George Beard, to describe a condition of profound nervous exhaustion (Beard 1869). The illness was characterised by mental and physical fatigue which could be exacerbated on the slightest exertion. A French doctor in the 1880s explained how even simple activities such as standing, talking or walking were problematic for his patient:

Her head was continually heavy [*alourdie*], the only thing she wants is to remain in bed. Any activity causes her the greatest fatigue. In the months preceding my first visit she had renounced all activity, and normally did not leave her bed at all. She said that her illness had begun with a great sense of weariness in the head, followed almost immediately by great muscular fatigue.

(Cheron 1893 cited in Shorter 1994)

Recent doctors' accounts of CFS are almost indistinguishable from such descriptions of neurasthenic patients. In his book *The Body at War*, John Dwyer (1988) provides a detailed account of Carol's battle with fatigue:

Her body was that of a very old woman she thought. It protested that it did not want to move; it was exhausted. More than that, it ached from head to toe. She could feel each muscle protesting even as she lay immobile in bed. Many of the muscles felt tender to her touch. With the maximum amount of will power she dragged her new self to the bathroom, then collapsed back on her bed, utterly exhausted from this effort. She had been tired before but never had she felt anything approaching this sensation. Her head was pounding and she recalls how confused she was.

(Dwyer 1988:192)

Like CFS, neurasthenia was associated with numerous other somatic complaints including headaches, general weakness, heart palpitations, gastrointestinal discomfort and muscle pain (Wessely 1990). As any form of exertion was seen to exacerbate the condition, rest was the advocated cure. In advising how to deal with neurasthenia it was stressed that 'any unnecessary expenditure of energy, must be averted, any superfluous task, any wasting of force' (Hartenberg cited in Shorter 1992:226). This advice is not dissimilar to the 'aggressive rest therapy' frequently prescribed for CFS sufferers in self-help manuals.

The controversy raised by neurasthenia was remarkably similar to that of the 1980s' 'yuppie flu' debate. Despite affirming that there were no physical signs of the disorder and that neurasthenia was compatible with the appearance of good health, Beard was adamant about the organic nature of the condition. He observed that the illness was most prevalent in the upper echelons of the community and concluded that neurasthenia was a physical response to the demands of industrialised society. In his view, over-exertion resulted in loss of nerve strength from nerves losing their natural charge. However, as with modern-day CFS, not everyone wholeheartedly accepted neurasthenia as an organic disorder. Indeed, many neurasthenics complained that they were treated with indifference by the medical profession (Wessely 1990). Despite this early scepticism, neurasthenia acquired credibility as a neurological condition and was a popular diagnosis in the early part of the twentieth century not only in the US, but as far afield as Europe and East Asia (Ware and Kleinman 1992).

In fact neurasthenia became so popular for a while that it was used to describe almost any complaint that included subjective symptoms (Shorter 1992). However, the early part of the twentieth century brought about a new sophistication in psychiatric classification or nosology. With this came the realisation that many patients previously labelled as neurasthenic were suffering from any of a wide range of disorders. Henri Feuillade in 1924 described how under the label of neurasthenia 'one finds melancholics, patients with compulsive thoughts [*des scrupeleux*], the anxious, the obsessed, the phobic, the impulsive, the degenerate, even some cases of neurosyphilis in remission' (cited in Shorter 1992:231).

This increasing recognition of distinct psychiatric disorders, together with the advent of Freudian ideology and psychodynamic theories of emotion, meant that ideas about neurasthenia began to shift from neurology to psychology (Greenberg 1990; Wessely 1990). Physicians began to focus on the analysis of unconscious conflict in chronically fatigued patients. Chronic fatigue was seen as misdirected neurotic energy or the unconscious expression of underlying emotional conflict (Greenberg 1990). People with neurasthenic symptoms became known as neurotic or hysterical and neurasthenia as originally described by Beard was rarely diagnosed. Today, neurasthenia no longer appears in recent editions of the *Diagnostic and Statistical Manual of Mental Disorders* (DSM). While it is retained in the section on Mental and Behavioural Disorders in the tenth revision of the *International Classification of Diseases* (ICD-10), it is classified under 'other neurotic disorders' and is largely regarded as a 'waste basket category' that can result in the missed diagnosis of depression or other medical conditions (David and Wessely 1993; Lee 1994). Thus, until the re-emergence of CFS as a unique disease of the 1980s, chronic fatigue became an 'invisible' diagnosis for the greater part of this century (Ware 1992).

War-related fatigue syndromes

Fatigue syndromes occurring during or after active combat also attracted attention at the turn of the century (Greenberg 1990; Hyams, Wignall and Roswell 1996). At the same time that ideas about neurasthenia were being formulated, another American physician described a very similar disease episode afflicting soldiers of the American Civil War, which he labelled 'irritable heart' (Da Costa 1871). The illness usually began with gastrointestinal upset followed by functional impairment aggravated by symptoms of exertional fatigue, disturbed sleep, dizziness, shortness of breath and sudden palpitations. Da Costa's emphasis on the last three symptoms suggests a substantial overlap with contemporary descriptions of panic and anxiety disorders. It is possible that some of the other symptoms reflected malnutrition, infections, stress or exhaustion. However, like neurasthenia, there were no consistent biological signs of disease and most irritable heart patients appeared to be in reasonable health. Da Costa believed the illness to be either of infectious origin or related to strenuous military duties. Treatment involved removal from active service and administration of a variety of tonics and medications for the heart (Demitrack and Abbey 1996).

A similar syndrome was common during World War I. This illness, referred to as the Da Costa syndrome, effort syndrome, and soldier's heart, incorporated most of the somatic symptoms described by Da Costa as well as a range of neuropsychological symptoms, such as forgetfulness and poor concentration (Greenberg 1990; Hyams *et al.* 1996). In many cases the symptoms were deemed serious enough to evacuate soldiers back to England. Effort syndrome was initially attributed to cardiac hypertrophy caused by over-exertion, but as the war progressed the illness was linked to a number of causes, including a past history of nervousness or physical weakness, infections and exhaustion. Cardiac medication was found to be ineffective for these patients and attributing their illness to heart disease appeared to hinder recovery and return to the trenches (Hyams *et al.* 1996). However, structured rehabilitation programmes incorporating a gradual return to exercise were found to be effective. By the end of the war it became accepted that effort syndrome was not caused exclusively by wartime exposure, but whether the illness was primarily physiological or psychological in origin was still uncertain (Hyams *et al.* 1996).

Effort syndrome remained a popular diagnosis at the beginning of World War II. However, attitudes towards the illness changed during the

1940s when Paul Wood, a distinguished British cardiologist, conducted a series of studies on a large group of patients with the syndrome in an attempt to discover whether the illness was primarily psychological or physical in nature. From this research, he concluded that premorbid and concurrent psychological factors were largely responsible for the generation of symptoms. He stated that ' patients should be informed of their illness, and treated as psychoneurotic; their distaste for this label may prove quite helpful ... The patient must be induced to believe he is suffering from the effects of emotional disturbance, and not from any disease or alteration of visceral function' (Wood 1941).

It is not hard to comprehend why a diagnosis which then held these connotations would prove to be less popular with patients. The disdain for the diagnosis appears to be reflected in the Korean and Vietnam wars, where fatigue-like illnesses were not reported as major medical problems, and what might previously have been labelled effort syndrome or soldier's heart, became known as battle fatigue, acute combat stress reaction, or post-traumatic stress disorder (Hyams *et al.* 1996).

Thus, fatigue-related war syndromes followed a similar path to neurasthenia. Faced with conditions that were more than likely multifactorial in nature, the medical profession chose to dispense with any evidence of physical disorder and to place the syndromes squarely in the psychiatric basket. As we will discuss in more detail in Chapter 3, this need to explain illnesses as either organic or psychiatric plagued much of the early research in CFS.

It is also notable that like neurasthenia, war-related fatigue syndromes have re-emerged in the past decade as the latest twentieth century disease: Gulf War syndrome. Gulf War syndrome was the label given to a series of symptoms reported by American, Canadian and British troops on returning home from the Persian Gulf war. These symptoms are almost identical to those of CFS and include fatigue, unrefreshing sleep, forgetfulness, headache, muscle pain, joint stiffness and sleep disturbance (Hyams *et al.* 1996). Large epidemiological studies have shown that when compared to other cohorts of soldiers, Gulf war soldiers certainly do report higher rates of symptoms and poorer health perceptions (Gray *et al.* 1999; Unwin *et al.* 1999). However, this appears to be a quantitative rather than a qualitative difference, as Gulf war soldiers' symptom profiles do not appear to be different from those of other soldiers (Ismail *et al.* 1999). No characteristic physical sign or laboratory abnormality has been linked to the syndrome (Gray *et al.* 1999; Hyams 1998a). These findings suggest that, despite popular belief that the illness is an immune-related disorder resulting from multiple allergies or chemical sensitivities, it may not be a unique syndrome (Wessely 1997).

Epidemic outbreaks of fatigue-like illnesses

While the individual diagnosis of neurasthenia declined rapidly after World War I, at least twenty-three epidemic outbreaks of chronic fatigue-like illnesses occurred between 1934 and 1958, during the time of the polio epidemics (Henderson and Shelkov 1959). Outbreaks were reported in the United States, England, Iceland, Denmark, Germany, Australia, Greece and South Africa (Shafran 1991). The epidemics were reported under a variety of names including Royal Free disease, Icelandic disease, epidemic vegetative neuritis and acute infective encephalomyelitis (Shafran 1991). At the time of each epidemic, almost all the outbreaks were considered to be caused by some mysterious pathological agent reflected in both the British and American collective terms for the outbreaks – benign myalgic encephalomyelitis (Anonymous editorial 1956) and epidemic neuromyasthenia (Henderson and Shelkov 1959). In fact, myalgic encephalomyelitis or ME is still a popular term for CFS in many parts of the world and is retained in ICD-10 as a synonym for post-infectious fatigue syndrome (David and Wessely 1993). This is despite the fact that the striking feature of all the outbreaks was the stark contrast between the lack of laboratory findings and the intensity of the malaise and symptoms reported (Demitrack and Abbey 1996).

In 1970 a detailed analysis of the Royal Free epidemic and review of fifteen of the outbreaks concluded that these epidemics were psychosocial phenomena (McEvedy and Beard 1970a). Two causal mechanisms were proposed: mass psychogenic illness or altered perceptions of the medical community, or both. Psychogenic illnesses present as medical problems which are predominantly caused by psychological factors. Mass psychogenic illnesses commonly occur in closed communities, such as nurses' homes and schools, and are characterised by the dramatic spread of a group of presenting symptoms (Skelton and Pennebaker 1982). The features of the Royal Free epidemic were used to support the mass psychogenic hypothesis (McEvedy and Beard 1970a). The spread of the Royal Free epidemic was explosive, starting off with fewer than five cases in mid-July and within two weeks escalating to a hundred cases. The hospital closed at the end of July and when it reopened three months later over three hundred patients had been affected. The presentation of symptoms commonly associated with psychogenic illness, such as loss of sensation in the hands and feet and over-breathing, provided additional support for the mass psychogenic hypothesis.

In a minority of the epidemics the spread of the illness was less sensational, leading McEvedy and Beard (1970b) to propose a different mechanism: altered medical perceptions. Here, suspected cases of polio triggered a scare of a polio epidemic. As further illness was expected, the community may have become overly sensitive to reports of symptoms in general, leading to cases of illness being documented that might otherwise have gone unreported. The symptoms were more variable and less dramatic than those reported during the Royal Free epidemic, ranging from fatigue to nausea and vomiting. These are all common symptoms which may not be reported to doctors in other social circumstances. The process of how oversensitivity or hypervigilance to symptoms can lead to increased reports of illness is discussed in detail in Chapter 5. Such situations probably represented pseudo-epidemics, where the rates of illness are normal but are perceived to be exceptionally high. Interestingly, a recent investigation which compared employees at two state offices which had reported an outbreak of fatiguing illness with an office of employees which had not reported an outbreak, found equivalent levels of fatigue symptoms in all three offices (Shefer *et al.* 1997). These results lend support to the idea that certain outbreaks of fatigue-like illnesses are an artiefact of hypervigilance to symptom reporting, rather than a true reflection of an unknown disease.

Not everyone agreed with McEvedy and Beard's conceptualisations and a more recent review of the outbreaks suggested that the aetiology of these outbreaks was more heterogeneous than previously reported. In this review Briggs and Levine (1994) suggested that although excessive fatigue, myalgia, headache and low grade fever were common to all epidemics, there were marked differences in the reporting of neuro-psychological symptoms, lending support to the notion that multiple aetiological agents were responsible for the outbreaks.

With the demise of the polio epidemics, and possibly influenced in part by the suggestion of mass psychogenic illness, few epidemics of chronic fatigue have been reported since the 1960s. In 1984, however, an outbreak of chronic fatigue was reported in New Zealand in the small rural town of Tapanui (Poore, Snow and Paul 1984). The commonly experienced symptoms were tiredness, mood and sleep disturbances, headache, and joint or muscle pain. Men and women were affected equally and this fact, coupled with the absence of 'hysterical' type symptoms such as pseudo-paraesthesias or unexplained losses of sensation, argued against the mass hysteria hypothesis (Murdoch 1988). Using a case–control approach Poore and colleagues (1984) ruled out pollution and chemical contaminants as possible causes. They were also unable to find any serological evidence of infection, but concluded that the clinical presentation made an unidentified virus the most likely cause. As this was the first report of such an illness in the country the local name for chronic fatigue became Tapanui flu.

A 10-year follow-up of the Tapanui cohort showed that a high proportion of patients recovered from the illness, with most returning to premorbid levels of activity (Levine 1997). These data suggest that epidemic outbreaks of fatigue may well be qualitatively different from currently defined CFS. A review of prognostic studies of currently defined Chronic Fatigue and CFS demonstrated that less than ten per cent return to premorbid levels of functioning and the majority remain significantly impaired (Joyce, Hotopf and Wessely 1997). Another, better known, American outbreak occurred in Lake Tahoe, Nevada. In contrast to the New Zealand epidemic, the American investigators did find evidence of elevated antibody titres to Epstein–Barr Virus (EBV), leading to the suggestion that the outbreak may be a chronic version of infectious mononucleosis, commonly known as glandular fever (Holmes *et al.* 1987).

Post-infectious fatigue syndromes

Glandular fever was linked to persistent fatigue as long ago as 1948 (Isaacs 1948), although it took another twenty years before EBV was identified as a major cause of the illness (Henle, Henle and Diehl 1968). This discovery was followed by a series of reports in the seventies and eighties that serologic markers of EBV were associated with idiopathic ongoing fatigue (Demitrack and Abbey 1996; Shafran 1991; Shorter 1992). Much of the recent interest in CFS has been attributed to two of these reports which appeared in a prominent American journal (Jones *et al.* 1985; Straus *et al.* 1985) and to the findings from the Lake Tahoe epidemic. As such, when the distinct possibility of an organic aetiology re-emerged, the recognition of chronic fatigue as a distinct diagnostic entity once again became popular.

It is noteworthy that these reports of chronic EBV infection made no reference to earlier prospective research which reported that both delayed recovery from glandular fever and the emergence of clinical features following EBV infection are linked to psychological factors (Kasl, Evans and Niederman 1979). Indeed, such findings were not only restricted to glandular fever. In a series of impressive prospective studies Imboden and colleagues demonstrated that ongoing symptoms from other acute infections such as influenza and brucellosis were largely dependent on psychological factors (Imboden, Canter and Cluff 1961; Imboden *et al.* 1959). These authors interpreted their results as suggesting that viral infections trigger depressive symptoms in psychologically vulnerable individuals. The clinical symptoms of depression become intertwined with the symptoms of acute infection, resulting in the experience of ongoing symptoms which patients often attribute to their initial viral infection. For quite some time prior to Imboden's studies, chronic malaise following illnesses such as brucellosis and influenza were thought to result from ongoing infection (see Demitrack and Abbey 1996 for review).

In summary, organic theories of chronic fatigue-like illnesses over the past century have ranged from reactions to stressors of modern society, physical over-exertion, effects of pollutants and infectious agents. Psychological theories have incorporated hysteria, neuroses, psychogenic illness and hypervigilance to symptom reporting. In all likelihood fatigue syndromes are heterogeneous in origin. For instance, in war-related syndromes some cases may represent anxiety and panic disorders. In other cases the promise of removal from the combat situation may promote the emergence or exaggeration of symptoms. The experience of stress, poor diet and exposure to foreign infectious agents may also cause some of the symptoms classified under war-related fatigue syndromes. In many cases a number of these factors may be relevant. For instance, the combination of the physical factors such as malnourishment and psychological factors such as anxiety could produce the composite of symptoms. However, it is evident from this historical account that medicine has generally been intolerant of a multifactorial approach. Mind–body dualism underscores the cycle of emergence of chronic fatigue as a distinct diagnostic entity (Ware 1993). The illness has either been conceptualised as physical or functional, only becoming popular once the respectability of organicity has been bestowed upon it. Inherent within this thinking is the twentieth-century attitude that a person with a physical diagnosis is more worthy of empathy and understanding than a person with a psychiatric diagnosis. A diagnosis of psychiatric disorder means that patients are often saddled with labels such as hysterical or neurotic, and worse still, lazy, incompetent or malingering. It is not hard to understand why an organic label is preferable. Thus, the very existence of fatigue syndromes has to a large extent been defined by culturally distinct illness beliefs (Ware and Kleinman 1992). A more detailed overview of these and other sociocultural factors in CFS is presented in Chapter 4.

The ultimate challenge for CFS will be its ability to flout history by remaining a diagnostic entity. Is this likely to happen? Simon Wessely and Arthur Kleinman suggest that it may, as in many ways CFS seems to be symbolic of a major paradigm shift in modern medicine, where researchers are slowly being forced to cross interdisciplinary boundaries (Kleinman 1993; Wessely 1995a). It is becoming increasingly difficult to ignore the relevance of both psychological and organic findings in CFS, and the ability to view CFS as a biopsychosocial phenomenon may well ensure its survival. Another shift which may influence the continued existence of CFS is the modern patient–doctor relationship (Wessely 1995a). While historical accounts have shown that the existence of fatigue-like illnesses has depended on medical decisions regarding the nature of the condition, the balance of power nowadays has shifted towards the patient (Shorter 1995). Academic arguments about the status of CFS have largely been overtaken by radical CFS self-help groups, who publish their own journals and have numerous talk groups on the internet (Davison and Pennebaker 1997). It is unlikely that these patients will allow the medical profession to delegitimise their condition or to forget about the organic features of the illness.

Chapter 2

Contemporary chronic fatigue syndrome

A unique entity?

As mentioned in Chapter 1, the renewed interest in chronic fatigue-like illnesses in the 1980s brought with it a confusing array of illness labels and definitions. This factor, coupled with the heterogeneous nature of fatigue syndromes, made it difficult to compare and evaluate research findings or draw any conclusions about the clinical nature of the condition. To address this problem, in 1987 the CDC in Atlanta convened a working party of American infectious disease and immunology specialists to develop standardised diagnostic criteria for the illness. This chapter reviews this and the subsequent definitions of CFS and discusses their limitations. In particular, the constraints related to the nature of fatigue and the overlap between CFS and other disorders are addressed. Finally, the epidemiology of the condition and the impact of CFS on both the individual and society are discussed.

Understanding the definitions of CFS is important for a number of reasons. First, it provides an indication of the clinical nature of CFS, particularly in terms of the type of fatigue experienced by these patients. Second, understanding the controversies surrounding the definition of the disorder provides some insight into the challenges researchers face. As you will observe in the following two chapters, discerning the causes of the illness is an important patient concern. However, the fact that the disorder is heterogeneous and has a number of definitions makes the process of interpreting results from causal studies very complex. Further, the overlap between CFS and other conditions raises issues about the application of the current classification of CFS. Undoubtedly it is useful for research purposes, but from a clinical point of view, understanding the broader group of syndromes of which CFS may form a part is equally significant. In the final section of this chapter the differences between medically defined CFS and patient defined CFS are discussed. This is a crucial concept in terms of understanding some of the psychological mechanisms of the disorder which are addressed in detail in Chapters 5–7.

Contemporary case definitions

The American definition

A primary task of the formative American working party was to decide on an appropriate name for the condition. CFS was unanimously agreed upon as it describes the central symptom of the disorder while avoiding assumptions about aetiology (Holmes *et al.* 1988). The name was less well received by the sufferers of the illness, epitomised by one patient's lament:

> The new name 'Chronic Fatigue Syndrome' is far too benign. It trivialises. How seriously would you take something called 'Chronic Thirst Syndrome'? And yet, diabetes is a very serious condition. 'Disabling Fatigue and Immune Dysfunction Syndrome' does a bit better; while more research should allow something more specific.
>
> (Thompson 1992:27)

This preference for a label which emphasises the pathophysiology or biological aspects of the illness is evident in much of the CFS self-help literature. Consequently, names such as chronic fatigue immune dysfunction syndrome (CFIDS) and myalgic encephalomyelitis (ME) still persist in the popular press and patients' self-help organisations. In fact in New Zealand, the national patient support organisation is called the Australian and New Zealand Myalgic Encephalomyelitis Society (ANZMES).

Despite this patient protest, as we discuss further in Chapter 3, there is no definitive clinical test available to diagnose CFS or to confirm its aetiology. The CDC working party, therefore, developed a definition based on a distinct symptom profile and the careful exclusion of known medical and psychiatric entities which could mimic the symptoms of CFS. The cardinal symptom for diagnosing CFS was described as persistent or debilitating fatigue which is new in origin, has been present for at least six months, does not resolve with bed-rest, and substantially reduces premorbid daily activity levels by 50 per cent (Holmes *et al.* 1988). In addition, eleven symptom criteria and three physician documented physical signs such as a low grade fever were specified as being integral to CFS. Patients needed to report at least eight of the eleven symptoms, or six of the symptoms together with two observable physical signs. Exclusionary illnesses included a wide range of medical conditions such as cancers and neuromuscular, endocrine and infectious diseases as well any current or past history of chronic psychiatric disorder.

This definition emphasised the presentation of physical signs and shortly after publication was found to be an inadequate and overly restrictive description of CFS. Manu, Lane and Mathews (1988) tested these criteria on 135 chronically fatigued patients. Only six subjects fulfilled the criteria for CFS and 91 had one or more psychiatric disorders felt to be the major cause of fatigue. They concluded that CFS, as defined, is uncommon even among patients with chronic fatigue. The inclusion of multiple somatic or physical symptoms seemed particularly problematic. It preferentially included patients with psychiatric complaints, who were in fact ineligible for diagnosis on exclusion criteria (Katon and Russo 1992). Further, it is difficult to substantiate that the presence of psychiatric disorders, such as depression or anxiety, fully accounts for the clinical presentation of CFS, as they may well be a result of the disabling illness. In response to these criticisms a group of researchers from the National Institute of Health proposed that the CDC criteria be revised to include certain comorbid or co-occurring psychiatric conditions such as nonpsychotic depressive, somatoform and anxiety disorders (Schluederberg *et al.* 1992).

The British definition

Also in response to criticisms of the original CDC definition, a multidisciplinary team of British researchers met in Oxford to rework CFS guidelines for research (Sharpe *et al.* 1991). The central criteria for disabling chronic fatigue were maintained, with the caveat that the fatigue must be both physical and mental. The presence of additional somatic symptoms was de-emphasised in an attempt to move away from thinking about CFS as an infective or immune process. Post-infectious fatigue syndrome (PIFS) was separated out as a subgroup of CFS. To be diagnosed with PIFS, laboratory evidence that infection had occurred at onset was necessary.

The Australian definition

At much the same time that the CDC definition was being formulated, Andrew Lloyd and his colleagues proposed an Australian definition

(Lloyd *et al.* 1988b). Like the British researchers, they concurred with the CDC label for the condition and the major fatigue criteria. They also agreed with the British group that additional physical symptoms were not essential for diagnosis, but patients had to report either difficulties with their concentration and memory or demonstrate abnormal cell-mediated immunity. The Australian definition differed, therefore, from both other definitions by specifying a laboratory marker, immune dysfunction, in the diagnosis.

Lloyd *et al.* (1988b) have been criticised for prematurely including this laboratory marker in their definition, as immune findings have been shown to be extremely variable across CFS groups, and the clinical significance of immune variables is unclear (Demitrack and Abbey 1996). Further, a study which compared the American, British and Australian case definitions found that similar immune abnormalities were found in groups meeting each of the three definitions, as well as in fatigued patients who met none of the case definitions (Bates *et al.* 1994). Immune findings are therefore unable to define a specific group of patients and do not add value to the current definition. It is, however, worth noting that when comparing the three case definitions, percentages of patients identified as having CFS are relatively similar and about two-thirds of patients met all three definitions (Bates *et al.* 1994). These findings are encouraging as they suggest that studies which have used individual case definitions are largely comparable.

A new consensus definition

In 1994 the CDC once again revised the criteria, this time including researchers from both Britain and Australia in the working party and from a wider background of professional disciplines (Fukuda *et al.* 1994). These criteria are summarised in Table 2.1. The presence of physical signs was dropped from the definition, and the number of unexplained somatic symptoms necessary for diagnosis was reduced from eight to four. A separate category, labelled idiopathic chronic fatigue, was created to describe patients who met the fatigue criteria without experiencing all the additional somatic complaints. The revised CDC criteria also stressed the heterogeneous nature of the condition and the need to investigate subgroups of CFS patients. They recommended that patients be subgrouped according to coexisting psychiatric conditions, levels and duration of fatigue, and current levels of disability.

Table 2.1 The 1994 CDC criteria for diagnosing CFS

1 *Presence of persistent or relapsing chronic fatigue which:*

- has been present for at least 6 months;
- is of new or definite onset;
- is not substantially alleviated by rest;
- results in substantial reduction in premorbid levels of occupational, educational, social, and/or personal activities.

2 *Four or more of the following symptoms, all of which must have occurred during at least six months of the illness and must not have predated the fatigue:*

- self-reported impairment in memory and concentration;
- sore throat;
- tender cervical or axillary lymph nodes;
- muscle pain;
- multi-joint pain;
- headaches of a new type;
- unrefreshing sleep;
- post-exertional malaise lasting more than 24 hours.

3 *Exclusionary criteria include:*

- any active medical condition which could explain chronic fatigue including untreated hypothyroidism, sleep apnoea, narcolepsy and iatrogenic conditions;
- any previously diagnosed medical condition whose resolution has not been documented beyond reasonable doubt and whose continued activity may explain the presence of chronic fatigue such as malignancies and unresolved hepatitis;
- any past or current history of psychotic major depression, bipolar affective disorder, schizophrenia, dementias, anorexia nervosa or bulimia nervosa;
- alcohol or other substance abuse within 2 years before the onset of the chronic fatigue and at any time afterwards.

(Adapted from Fukuda *et al.* 1994)

Validity issues: symptom counts and the nature of fatigue

In summary, CFS specialists have worked hard at developing effective diagnostic and research criteria for CFS and it is encouraging to see that researchers from different countries have managed to pool their ideas and work together at refining the definition. Despite these advancements, these criteria are purely descriptive and none of these definitions has particular validity. The core complaint of fatigue in CFS is based on subjective experience and to date there is no way of objectively validating this symptom (Wessely 1998). Whether or not additional somatic symptoms should be included as part of the definition is debatable. Wessely and colleagues, using a list of thirty-two somatic symptoms, demonstrated that all symptoms were rated significantly higher by chronic fatigue and CFS patients when compared to healthy controls (Wessely *et al.* 1996a). Symptoms included in the current definition were not specific to CFS and were highly correlated with psychiatric disorder. Hickie *et al.* (1995) found that CFS patients could be divided into two distinct groups based on symptom reports. The larger group, thought to be more typical of CFS patients, reported an average of four additional symptoms. The remaining one-third of patients reported a mean of twenty-four symptoms and may well be more representative of a primary somatisation disorder: a chronic psychiatric condition characterised by multiple physical complaints. Consequently, a maximum number of symptoms may be a more appropriate criterion than a minimum number.

Further, whether or not CFS is indeed a distinct clinical entity is debatable. A large survey of fatigue in the community found that cases of CFS fell at the severe end of the continuum of fatigue, without any clear or definite cut-off point (Pawlikowska *et al.* 1994). Studies which have compared patients with CFS and CF on measures of disability and distress find few differences except for the number of somatic complaints (Swanink *et al.* 1995; Wessely *et al.* 1996a; Zubieta *et al.* 1994). As such, the distinction between idiopathic chronic fatigue and CFS may well be somewhat arbitrary. In addition, the current criteria still incorporate a heterogeneous group of patients and, as we explain further in the following section, CFS overlaps significantly with a range of other conditions.

Overlapping syndromes

There is considerable overlap between CFS and psychiatric disorder, particularly depression. The relationship with psychiatric disorder is both controversial and complex and will be dealt with later in Chapter 4. However, there are a number of conditions such as fibromyalgia, chronic back or pelvic pain, multiple chemical sensitivities, irritable bowel syndrome, repetitive strain injury, migraine and tinnitus which, like CFS, present with medically unexplained aversive symptoms. The terms functional somatic syndrome (Barsky and Borus 1999; Wessely, Nimnuan and Sharpe 1999) or symptom based conditions (Hyams 1998b) have been used as a collective term for these conditions. Functional somatic syndromes are characterised by a degree of suffering and disability that appears to be out of proportion with any observable pathophysiology (Barsky and Borus 1999). Although each of these syndromes is defined in terms of a specific symptom profile, fatigue and/or muscle pain, or spasm, are key presenting symptoms in almost all of them. Other common symptoms include sleep difficulties, problems with memory and concentration, gastrointestinal symptoms, shortness of breath and sore throat (Hyams 1998b). All of these symptoms have a high incidence in the general population and in Chapter 5 we talk more about the possible common mechanisms behind these symptom reports.

Psychiatric illness in functional somatic syndromes

In addition to presenting with overlapping symptoms, patients with functional somatic syndromes report substantially higher levels of psychiatric morbidity than patients with other medical conditions. For instance, about 60–70 per cent of patients with these conditions have had an episode of depression some time in their lives compared to 10–20 per cent of patients with other medical illnesses (Hudson and Pope 1994; Russo *et al.* 1994). Anxiety and somatisation disorders are also over-represented in these groups. Despite this overlay with psychiatric illness, patients with these syndromes often have a strong belief in the organic nature of their conditions and strongly resist information that challenges these beliefs (Barsky and Borus 1999).

Chronic fatigue syndrome and other functional syndromes

A handful of studies have made direct comparisons between CFS patients and those with other functional somatic syndromes. Fibromyalgia, a condition characterised by chronic musculoskeletal pain occurring at specific anatomical sites referred to as tender points, appears to have substantial overlap with CFS (Buchwald *et al.* 1987; Goldenberg *et al.* 1990; Buchwald and Garrity 1994). In fact, in many cases the disorders are indistinguishable with the majority of CFS patients meeting criteria for fibromyalgia and vice versa. Perhaps this is not surprising, as although the chief presenting complaint of fibromyalgia is pain at specific tender points, other key symptoms include fatigue, sleep disturbance, headache, depression and anxiety. Further, Buchwald and Garrity (1994) found that symptoms previously associated with CFS but not fibromyalgia, such as recurrent sore throat and low grade fevers, were reported by a substantial number of fibromyalgia patients. Similarly, Goldenberg and colleagues found that tender points which were previously thought to be unique to fibromyalgia were present in more than two-thirds of CFS patients (1990). Both groups report equivalent levels of sickness-related disability, with patients who meet criteria for both diagnoses being the most impaired (Buchwald 1996). Interestingly, although CFS is traditionally associated with beliefs about a viral onset, one study found that over half their sample of fibromyalgia patients made similar attributions (Buchwald 1996).

There is also substantial overlap between people diagnosed with multiple chemical sensitivities (MCS) and those with CFS. MCS is a disorder which is believed to be triggered by exposure to various chemicals at doses much lower than those expected to cause adverse effects in humans. Symptoms are recurrent and can involve many bodily systems. Although only 30 per cent of MCS patients meet full criteria for a diagnosis of CFS, compared to 70 per cent of fibromyalgia patients (Buchwald and Garrity 1994), 80 per cent of them meet all the CFS fatigue criteria. MCS patients also report similar levels of neuropsychological symptoms such as loss of memory and concentration (Buchwald and Garrity 1994; Fiedler *et al.* 1996). The key feature of MCS, adverse reactions to environmental agents, is reported by up to 63 per cent of CFS patients (Buchwald and Garrity 1994).

The results of these comparison studies suggest that diagnoses assigned to patients with CFS, fibromyalgia or MCS may well depend on their dominant complaint and health practitioner preference, rather than on actual illness process. For instance, a patient referred to a rheumatologist may be diagnosed with fibromyalgia, while the same patient referred to an infectious disease specialist may be diagnosed with CFS or post-viral fatigue syndrome. Similarly, a diagnosis of MCS may be more likely if the patient is referred to an occupational physician or decides to see a naturopath or homeopath. Who the patient decides to consult will also have a bearing on diagnosis and may well depend on the patient's beliefs about what caused their illness in the first place. For instance, a patient who dates the onset of their condition to chemical exposure will be more likely to be diagnosed with MCS than CFS. This patient may also be less inclined to consult an infectious disease specialist.

Further studies comparing CFS samples with other symptom-based conditions have found CFS patients demonstrate somewhat higher levels of psychopathology and disability. Blakely *et al.* (1991) and Russo *et al.* (1994) have reported striking similarities between CFS patients and groups with chronic pain, tinnitus and unexplained dizziness on measures of personality and psychopathology. However, the CFS patients displayed significantly higher levels of neuroticism, medically unexplained symptoms, and lifetime psychiatric diagnoses than the other patient groups. When compared to patients with irritable bowel syndrome, CFS patients not only had higher symptom reports and poorer psychological well-being, but they also reported lower levels of motivation and physical activity (Vercoulen *et al.* 1994) .

Explanations for the overlap in functional somatic syndromes

It is therefore hard to refute the substantial phenomenological overlap between CFS and a number of other functional somatic syndromes. What the overlap actually represents is more difficult to explain. It is worth mentioning that some of the observed similarities might be exaggerated by the fact that all the samples studied were drawn from tertiary care and may not be representative of individuals with these conditions in the general population. However, the extent and consistency of the association observed makes it implausible to suggest that the relationship is just coincidental or methodological. One possibility is that a modern trend has arisen which sees committees somewhat arbitrarily deciding on definitions and labels for what are essentially a single psychiatric entity or form of somatisation (Shorter 1995). Although somatisation is currently defined as a distinct disorder in the *Diagnostic and Statistical Manual for Mental Disorders* (DSM IV), proponents of this view suggest that somatisation is more accurately conceptualised as a dimensional construct (Barsky and Borus 1999; Wessely *et al.* 1999). Somatisation is viewed as a process by which common somatic sensations or symptoms of distress, or both, are incorrectly attributed to a serious disease or illness. When the psychological context of the symptoms is denied by both patient and practitioner, somatisation becomes labelled a disorder. Higher symptom counts and disability represent greater underlying distress, which would suggest that disorders such as CFS and fibromyalgia sit at the extreme end of the somatisation continuum. The relationship across groups between symptom reports and psychiatric disorder or psychological distress goes some way to providing support for this hypothesis (Russo *et al.* 1994).

Another possibility is that these functional somatic syndromes share a common underlying pathophysiology, which may occur along a spectrum of severity (Hudson and Pope 1994). This theory is derived in part from the observation that many of these disorders have been shown to respond to low doses of antidepressants (Gruber, Hudson and Pope 1996). However, neither the somatisation nor the pathophysiological explanations account for the differences between the idiopathic disorders, particularly in the dominant presenting symptom. While, as mentioned earlier, certain patients do meet more than one diagnosis and may be labelled according to physician bias, there are others who may more distinctly meet criteria for a specific condition such as tinnitus or migraine.

A study using confirmatory factor analysis of symptoms reported by patients consulting their general practitioner argues against these syndromes existing purely as a single entity (Kirmayer and Robbins 1991). A single somatisation factor was unable to account for the variation amongst symptoms. A five-factor solution which separated primary symptoms of fibromyalgia, irritable bowel syndrome, CFS, somatic anxiety and somatic depression appeared to be the best statistical solution. All five factors were highly correlated and pure types of the syndrome were less likely to occur than mixed types, suggesting that the syndromes do not occur in isolation. However, the results of this study still suggest that unique aetiological factors may contribute to the different presentations of these conditions.

It may be that certain of these conditions have unique pathophysiological underpinnings. In the following chapter we review the findings which suggest that there are physiological mechanisms associated with CFS. However, at this stage there is little evidence to show that these mechanisms are different from those of other functional syndromes. Even if distinct physiological concomitants are linked to individual conditions, it is unlikely that they will account for the extent of the disability experienced by these patients. In Chapters 5 and 6 we discuss in detail how symptom interpretation and illness beliefs may prove to be the common mechanisms linking these disorders together.

The epidemiology and impact of chronic fatigue syndrome

Although CFS may be part of a broad spectrum of disorders, the fact that we have definite diagnostic criteria for the illness means that it is possible to estimate how many people are afflicted with this disorder. In this final section we demonstrate that CFS, as currently defined, is not an uncommon illness. Perhaps the most important feature of the illness is not whether or not it is unique, but rather that it has a profound impact both on the individual and on society.

Epidemiology of chronic fatigue

Fatigue itself is one of the most commonly reported symptoms in the community, with about one-third of the population reporting symptoms of fatigue or exhaustion at any one time (Lewis and Wessely 1992). For around 18 per cent of the population the fatigue is considered chronic (Pawlikowska *et al.* 1994). Studies have consistently shown that there is a strong positive correlation between persistent fatigue and psychiatric morbidity (Lawrie and Pelosi 1995; Pawlikowska *et al.* 1994; Price *et al.* 1992). Age and social class appear to have little effect on fatigue symptoms, but there is a small gender bias (David *et al.* 1990; Lewis and Wessely 1992; Pawlikowska *et al.* 1994). Women are approximately 1.5 times more likely to experience fatigue than men (Lewis and Wessely 1992).

Fatigue severity is also associated with the explanations patients give for their fatigue. The most common attributions are psychosocial and people who make either family, social or emotional attributions have lower fatigue scores than those who relate their fatigue to physical factors (David *et al.* 1990; Lawrie and Pelosi 1995; Pawlikowska *et al.* 1994). A minority, who attribute their fatigue to a virus or CFS, have the highest fatigue scores of all. There are few gender differences in attributions, but women are much more likely than men to blame their fatigue on social factors such as family responsibilities, particularly caring for young children (David *et al.* 1990). It is possible that such social factors account for women reporting higher levels of fatigue. The fact that women have increased psychiatric morbidity does not appear to account for elevated fatigue levels (Pawlikowska *et al.* 1994).

Epidemiology of chronic fatigue syndrome

Chronic fatigue is therefore a common symptom experienced by people of all social classes. But what of the syndrome? The name 'yuppie flu' was based on the stereotype that the illness affected well-educated, overworked white people. Certainly, early reports suggested that CFS was indeed an illness of the white middle class (Komaroff and Buchwald 1991; Manu, Lane and Mathews 1993a). Women were three times more likely to be affected than men and certain professional groups, such as teachers and health professionals, were reported as being particularly at risk. However, these statistics were based on patients recruited from tertiary care, who quite often had made a self-diagnosis before requesting specialist treatment, and were clearly unrepresentative of all CFS cases. Patients who diagnose themselves with CFS and those who present to tertiary care are more likely to be better educated and to belong to the upper socio-economic classes than those presenting in primary care (Euga *et al.* 1996; Pawlikowska *et al.* 1994).

To address the problem of selection bias, more recent epidemiological studies have gathered their data from the community and from primary care samples. These studies have generally found that the social class and occupational distribution of CFS patients reflects that of the general population (Euga *et al.* 1996; Lawrie and Pelosi 1995; Lloyd *et al.* 1990; Wessely *et al.* 1997). Two studies have reported equal sex distributions for CFS patients (Lawrie and Pelosi 1995; Lloyd *et al.* 1990), although others still find a higher incidence in women (Euga *et al.* 1996; Gunn, Connell and Randall 1993; Wessely *et al.* 1997). However, this gender bias is less marked than originally reported and is not always significant. One factor that appears to be unaffected by whether data is collected from primary or tertiary care is the high level of psychopathology reported in CFS patients (McDonald *et al.* 1993b). Comorbid psychiatric disorder is an important consideration, as it is associated with a greater degree of functional impairment in CFS (Wessely *et al.* 1997).

Prevalence statistics for CFS have been influenced by methodology. Studies relying on sentinel physicians to identify cases of CFS retrospectively have estimated rates ranging between 2 and 130 per 100,000 population (Gunn *et al.* 1993; Ho-Yen and McNamara 1991; Lloyd *et al.* 1990). Problems of varied recognition of CFS between practitioners, poor response rates, and application of different definitions may have contributed to the discrepant findings. More recent studies using systematic case ascertainment suggest that these figures are conservative and that CFS is a far greater problem than originally thought. An American study comparing the three definitions reported a point prevalence of 0.3 per cent for the original CDC criteria, 0.4 per cent for the British criteria and 1.0 per cent for the Australian definition (Bates *et al.* 1993). A British study of over 2,000 adults recruited from primary care estimated an even higher prevalence rate of 2.6 per cent of the population using the new 1994 CDC criteria (Wessely *et al.* 1997). Of particular interest was the finding that only 12 per cent of people who met criteria for CFS actually labelled themselves as such. This is important not only because it highlights the role of selection bias in studies, but because a self- diagnosis is related to both higher levels of fatigue and psychological morbidity (Pawlikowska *et al.* 1994). In addition, as we will argue in Chapter 6, the fact that patients believe that they have CFS may well be a more important defining characteristic than whether or not they meet predetermined operational criteria for the condition.

Disability and prognosis in chronic fatigue syndrome

CFS has a marked impact on people's lives. Studies have shown that they report greater levels of dysfunction in almost all domains of life when compared to patients who have multiple sclerosis (MS), hypertension, congestive heart failure, type II diabetes mellitus, and acute myocardial infarction (Komaroff *et al.* 1996; Schweitzer *et al.* 1995). In fact, only terminally ill cancer and stroke patients are known to report equivalent levels of disability to CFS patients (Schweitzer *et al.* 1995). Approximately a quarter of all CFS patients describe themselves as regularly bedridden (Komaroff and Buchwald 1991), with around 40 per cent unemployed because of their illness and a further 20 to 30 per cent having to reduce their work commitments to part-time (Bombardier and Buchwald 1995; Lloyd *et al.* 1990).

Interviews with CFS patients provide a rich picture of just how profoundly the illness impacts on all aspects of their lives. One patient explains:

> It's changed absolutely everything I do: what I eat, where I live. It's stopped my life. My whole perception of life, which took 30 years to put together is totally gone.
>
> (cited in Anderson and Estwing Ferrans 1997:363)

Another patient illustrates the extent of the losses experienced by many CFS patients:

> I spend 21–23 hours of my day lying down. Even then, it's an effort to use parts of my body. To lift my hand to write a check is too much. Last time I tried walking, I got to the end of the block and had to lay down for 15 minutes before I had the strength to go back home. So I don't even consider anymore. I haven't dealt with problems that I'll eventually have to deal with: like my boyfriend leaving me, my lost job and friends ... these are awful things, but right now I have no stamina to think about them. All I care about is getting to a level where my illness is tolerable.
>
> (cited in Anderson and Estwing Ferrans 1997:363)

Not only does the illness affect people's ability to carry out daily tasks and to work, but it also devastates social activities and relationships. A patient elaborates:

> I couldn't ski or play volley ball anymore and friends of 15 years stopped returning my calls and quietly disappeared. I wasn't fun anymore.
>
> (cited in Anderson and Estwing Ferrans 1997:363)

Another young 14-year-old sufferer, Deirdre, finds that her friends view her CFS as a way of getting out of unpleasant commitments. In response to being told how lucky she is, Deirdre replies:

> Do they think I enjoy being sick? Enjoy not being able to play sport, or go to school camps, not being able to go on bikes, not being able to go to the late movies because I have to be in bed at night at 8.30, because if I'm not I won't be able to do anything the next day? ... They say they wish they could live like I do. How would they like being lonely all the time? Not having a really close friend except your family. They seem to think my life's a barrel of laughs. Well it's not. Why can't they understand?
>
> (Deirdre 1990:32)

For a substantial number of patients this disability continues for many years. A US study of CFS patients recruited from a range of geographic areas reported a mean length of illness of 7.2 years (Gunn *et al.* 1993).

Here in New Zealand, we found that a national sample of 233 patients, belonging to an ME support group, reported an average length of illness of 10.8 years (Moss-Morris, Petrie and Weinman 1996b). Patients meeting the full definition for CFS have a poorer prognosis than patients with Chronic Fatigue, reporting greater symptom severity and higher levels of psychopathology and disability (Joyce *et al.* 1997). Two prospective studies of the natural course of CFS over an 18-month period found that only 2 to 3 per cent of CFS patients report complete resolution of symptoms (Bombardier and Buchwald 1995; Vercoulen *et al.* 1996b). The number of patients reporting improvement over time varied, with the Dutch study finding that only 17 per cent of their patients had improved (Vercoulen *et al.* 1996b), compared to 61 per cent in the American study (Bombardier and Buchwald 1995). These differences may reflect the way in which improvement was measured. Only the Dutch study validated their improvement scale with other measures of symptoms and disability, as well as comparing improved patients with healthy subjects.

Undoubtedly the degree of disability in CFS is immense, but there are a number of other points that are worth noting in terms of understanding disability in CFS. First, despite this high morbidity, CFS is a low mortality illness with no reports of deaths linked directly to the condition (Joyce *et al.* 1997). Second, the degree of disability varies from person to person and the statistics show that some people manage to continue working. Patients also describe substantial daily variability. Third, although CFS patients report higher levels of disability than MS patients, objective measures of activity levels in these two groups have been shown to be equivalent (Vercoulen *et al.* 1997). Cognitive factors, such as the expectation that certain activities would cause fatigue, seem to play an important role in causing low activity levels in CFS patients but not MS patients. This suggests that self-reports of disability in CFS may differ from objective measures of disability. The role that illness beliefs play in the experience of subjective disability in this group will be dealt with further in Chapter 6.

The economic impact of CFS

The debilitating nature of CFS clearly results in substantial personal costs, but what of the economic implications? There are direct costs associated with the increased utilisation of health care resources, and the indirect costs incurred through cessation or reduction in employment (Lloyd and Pender 1992). The direct costs include consultations with general practitioners and specialists, which frequently generate a profusion of diagnostic tests and prescribed treatments. On average, CFS patients in Australia consult a general practitioner or specialist 18 times a year specifically for their CFS (Lloyd and Pender 1992). The total annual health care cost for one CFS patient amounts to approximately $A2,000. Patients also consult a range of alternative health care providers, such as naturopaths, osteopaths and acupuncturists. Individual patients in America have spent as much as $60,000 on dubious, unproven remedies for their CFS (Sullivan 1995).

The indirect costs of the illness are even higher, both to the individual in lost earnings and to the country in lost income tax and social security payments. Average income forgone by CFS patients in Australia was $A7,500 per year, which amounted to a tax revenue loss of $A1,700 (Lloyd and Pender 1992). Overall, the economic impact of CFS to the Australian government and the community is approximately $A9,500 per patient. If this cost is extrapolated to the conservative CFS prevalence rate in Australia (Lloyd *et al.* 1990), CFS costs the community $A59 million per annum. These economic estimates do not include the 13 per cent of patients who are mislabelled as having CFS (Lloyd *et al.* 1990), nor do they take into consideration that current estimates of CFS are ten-fold higher than the initial Australian estimate (Wessely *et al.* 1997).

There are also huge costs to private insurance agencies. A Canadian study examined the long-term disability claims due to CFS and fibromyalgia. Together these illnesses represented 302 claims producing monthly payments of $291,000 (Cameron 1995). The major difficulty for insurance companies is that the causes of CFS are still hotly debated and there are few reliable and objective methods for assessing the severity of the condition. In the following two chapters, we will provide an overview of the causal theories of CFS and a review of the literature which supports or refutes these ideas.

In summary, conceptualising CFS is not straightforward and can include a number of different dimensions. The medical profession has provided definite diagnostic criteria for the condition. This is an important step in standardising research of this condition, but many patients who meet diagnostic criteria for the illness do not identify themselves as such, while others who do not meet criteria believe they have the illness. The belief that one has CFS appears to be one of the most important factors in predicting disability in this illness. Another argument is that CFS is not a distinct illness, but rather that it falls on the extreme end of a continuum of fatigue. It also overlaps with a number of other medically unexplained conditions which may all form part of a single entity called functional somatic syndromes. Aside from the academic debate of how best to define the illness, CFS is definitely a significant public health problem, affecting up to 2.6 per cent of the population. From a clinical point of view the most important feature of the illness is that it has extremely distressing consequences for individuals, often rendering them severely disabled for lengthy periods of time.

Chapter 3

Chronic fatigue syndrome as a biomedical illness

Objective findings and the patient's perspective

Theories of CFS which incorporate biological, psychological and social aspects of the illness have evolved in the past few years. However, it is difficult to appreciate these without first exploring the findings which have emerged from each of these fields. This chapter provides an overview of the progression of CFS research in the biomedical field. We have already seen that the re-emergence and popularity of CFS centred on the acknowledgement of the organic nature of the condition. The initial enthusiasm for viral theories has to a large extent been superseded by immunological and central nervous system (CNS) or brain hypotheses of the disorder. Ideas about pollutants and allergies still abound in the popular CFS literature, while investigators are forming new hypotheses such as CFS being a disorder of sleep, breathing problems, or low blood pressure. The evidence for each of these hypotheses is briefly reviewed together with examples of patients' ideas and beliefs about the various causes of their illness and some of their reactions to the research findings. The implications of CFS patients' causal beliefs will be discussed further in later chapters.

Viral findings

Most CFS patients seen in tertiary clinics predate the onset of their condition to an acute infective episode (Komaroff and Buchwald 1991; Lloyd *et al.* 1990; Wessely and Powell 1989). This is not altogether surprising as CFS shares a number of qualities with viral illnesses such as a sudden onset, fatigue, muscle aches and pains and fuzzy headedness. A CFS patient explains on an internet chat group:

> When I am feeling least well, I tend to have a prickly throat, like a

mild sore throat. So I feel that a virus is at the root of my problem, which started 5 years ago with a conventional cold and sore throat, from which I have never recovered. Most of the time I feel as if I have 'flu: body aches and pains and severe fatigue. I don't know what is the mechanism by which the 'flu virus produces these feelings in normal individuals. But my strong suspicion is that it is this mechanism which is at the root of my CFS.

A medical doctor and sufferer of CFS, describes the onset of his illness while on a family holiday:

> I was extremely fit physically, and played a strenuous game of tennis regularly. My family and I had no psychiatric history. In particular, I had never suffered with depression. I developed what at the time seemed to be a minor upper respiratory tract infection. The only unusual symptom, which I had never had with previous viral infections, was muscle aches in my legs. In retrospect, I feel this was a very significant symptom as I believe the virus was causing damage centrally while manifesting peripherally in the muscle. This is my own personal belief which is based on my symptoms and not on any scientific fact.
>
> (Lopis 1995:16)

For some patients the virus is seen not only to trigger the condition but to perpetuate it as well. One patient divulges:

> I think it is a virus … And what I explained to the doctor was that there was a feeling that there was a virus in my body that was dormant for, you know, a good bit of the time, and then all of a sudden would come out to the fore, and come out to the surface every now and then.
>
> (cited in Ax, Greg and Jones 1997:251)

Retrospective studies

In response to patients' reports researchers have worked hard to pin down the elusive pathogen. They have investigated the possible role of herpesviruses including EBV, cytomegalovirus (CMV) and human herpesvirus 6 (HHV6); enteroviruses: largely coxsackie B; retroviruses such as human T cell leukaemia virus type 2 (HTLV-2) and the spumaviruses; *Borrelia burgdoferi* and Borna disease virus. As it is difficult to measure directly the presence of a virus, most of these studies have relied on the presence of elevated antibodies in the body. Antibodies are assumed to reflect the body's immune response to the presence of a viral or bacterial infection. Although some studies have reported elevated levels of viral antibodies in groups of CFS patients the results are inconsistent and there is often considerable overlap between CFS patients and controls (Ablashi 1994; Hotchin *et al.* 1989; Kawai and Kawai 1992; Landay *et al.* 1991; Levy 1994; MacDonald *et al.* 1996).

A large study which tested for antibodies to thirteen viruses found that none of these could either discriminate CFS patients from healthy controls, or CFS patients who reported a viral onset from those who did not (Buchwald *et al.* 1996). Other studies compared CFS patients with and without evidence of EBV and found that there was no difference in clinical presentation and outcome between these two groups (Hellinger *et al.* 1988; Mathews, Lane and Manu 1991). Finally, Straus and colleagues (1988a) tested the effectiveness of Acyclovir, an antiviral drug, in a randomised controlled trial of CFS patients. They were unable to demonstrate any clinical efficacy for the drug, with clinical improvement more likely to be correlated with improved psychological status than changes in the immune system. Thus, it has become increasingly apparent that viral antibodies have little diagnostic or prognostic value in CFS.

One of the reasons some CFS groups may demonstrate elevated levels of antibodies is that the presence of antibodies can reflect differences in psychological states. For instance, EBV has been implicated in depression, and elevated antibody titres to EBV in healthy people have been shown to indicate high levels of stress (Moss-Morris 1997a). In these situations, elevated titres reflect a possible immune response to psychological factors rather than a viral infection.

Prospective studies

The viral studies mentioned so far have all been retrospective in design in that they investigated patients who already had CFS. To rule out convincingly the role of viruses in CFS, we need to turn to prospective studies. These studies investigate causes by studying people before they contract the illness of interest. Two prospective studies have shown that common viral infections, such as upper respiratory tract infections, are not associated with the subsequent development of either chronic fatigue or CFS (Cope *et al.* 1994; Wessely *et al.* 1995b).

Nonetheless, there is some evidence that certain severe infections may play a role in select cases of CFS. Acute hepatitis and glandular fever have both been shown to be risk factors for the development of ongoing fatigue six months or more after initial infection (Berelowitz *et al.* 1995; White *et al.* 1995), although viral meningitis, an infection of the membranes surrounding the brain and spinal cord, has not (Hotopf, Noah and Wessely 1996).

Severe infections, however, cannot explain the majority of CFS cases. Fewer than 1 per cent of patients are able to pre-date their chronic fatigue to hepatitis and of those who do develop post-hepatitis fatigue, only 4 per cent attribute this to CFS (Berelowitz *et al.* 1995). On the surface it appears that the viral findings are in stark contrast to the prevalent reports from patients that their CFS began with a viral infection. Nevertheless, two possibilities exist, not necessarily mutually exclusive, for the role of viruses in CFS. First, viruses may be precipitating events which interact with psychosocial factors in developing CFS. Second, viruses could act as a precipitant for immune abnormalities in vulnerable individuals. While the virus itself is eliminated, the immune system is unable to return to its normal balance (Levy 1994). The following section deals with issues related to this second hypothesis, while the first hypothesis will be discussed in detail in Chapter 6.

Immunological findings

The support for immune theories of CFS is clearly illustrated in one of the preferred patient names for CFS, Chronic Fatigue and Immune Dysfunction Syndrome or CFIDS. The patient organisation in the USA uses this term and has a regular journal entitled *The CFIDS Chronicle*. The metaphor of a defence system that has gone awry is a common theme in the patient literature. One self-help journal reports that 'The typical CFIDS immune system is "noisy" or overactive, churning out chemicals in a chronic war against a real or perceived invader' (*Meeting-Place* 1996:23). A similar theme is evident not only in the content, but in the title of a book on CFS called *The Body at War* (Dwyer 1988).

Patients also make the comparison with other disorders where the immune system is severely compromised. In a recent study one of our CFS participants wrote:

Chronic Fatigue is an infliction equal in severity to some major physical disabilities. People with such severe disabilities can often be
happier in life and derive greater enjoyment than others not so in-
flicted yet suffering from CFS. I believe CFS is related to a breakdown in the immune system. Strange that this link is similar to the
problem facing AIDS.

The role of the immune system in CFS is most commonly conceptualised by patients as a reaction to certain trigger factors such as a virus,
allergens or stress. This model is clearly illustrated by a patient who told
us that prior to the onset of her CFS she had a particularly stressful few
years in terms of her personal relationships. She went on to explain:

I was working in a fairly high stress job and also trying to achieve
things in my life such as having a house built etc – all extremely high
stress situations. I believe the combination of these things seriously
affected my immune system and although my sickness appeared as a
viral illness which my immune system couldn't cope with I feel the
background to it all definitely was stress – emotional and physical.

The effects of past immunisations on the immune system have also
received bad press in the past few years. Mary, an ex-nurse, writes:

My illness began when my immune system was compromised by
immunisations and vaccinations during my nursing training 1950
onwards, culminating in total physical breakdown in 1983.

(Richards 1991:51)

So for a number of CFS patients, the immune hypothesis makes sense.
The CFS research in this area, however, is a bit more confusing. In interpreting the results, it helps to have some understanding of the functioning of the immune system. Put simply, the immune system protects the
body from potentially harmful organisms, such as viruses and bacteria,
which are collectively referred to as antigens. The cells of the immune
system operate in two ways in this process: first by destroying invading
antigens which is a function of the body's *innate immunity*, and second
through *acquired immunity*, which includes the formation of specific
antibodies and sensitised lymphocytes or white blood cells which can
destroy antigens. Acquired immunity can be divided into humoral
(blood) and cellular processes. Although these processes operate in an

integrated fashion, for ease of interpretation the results from CFS immune studies are discussed under these headings.

Humoral immune studies

Humoral immunity is mediated by lymphocytes or white blood cells known as B cells. The B cells are responsible for producing antigen-specific antibodies known as immunoglobins. In other words, when your body is attacked by a virus, an immunoglobin that is specific to that particular virus will be produced by the B cells. These immunoglobins attach to the surface of antigens in an effort to neutralise or destroy them before they affect the cells of the body. B cells also give rise to memory cells which protect against further infection by the specific antigen. The elevated antibody findings discussed in the viral section provide some evidence for altered humoral activity in CFS. Elevations in specific subsets of B cells have also been reported by some investigators, although most studies have been unable to demonstrate differences in the overall numbers of B cells (Buchwald and Komaroff 1991; Gupta and Vayuvegula 1991; Klimas *et al.* 1990; Tirelli *et al.* 1994). Both decreases and increases in immunoglobin subclasses have been reported, but a recent study on a larger group of CFS patients found no evidence for these alterations (Bennett *et al.* 1996). Finally, increased circulating immune complexes have been found in CFS populations (Bates *et al.* 1995; Natelson *et al.* 1995). Overall, the findings are small and inconsistencies exist across studies. Nonetheless, there is sufficient evidence to suggest a mild form of non-specific immune activation in some CFS patients (Krupp and Pollina 1996).

Cellular immune studies

Cellular immunity is mediated predominantly by T cell lymphocytes which promote humoral immune functions and destroy altered cells of the body such as those infected by viruses. T cells are divided into a number of groups each with a specific function, including natural killer (NK) cells and cytotoxic T cells which directly attack altered cells, memory T cells which remain after infection to defend against a recurrence, helper T cells which stimulate the production of both humoral and cellular white blood cells, and suppressor T cells which slow down or stop the immune processes.

T cell counts

Cell counts are often an indicator of compromise to the immune system. For instance, one of the features of Acquired Immune Deficiency Syndrome (AIDS) is a drop in the number of T cells which means fewer cells are available to fight infection and to simulate the production of white blood cells. There is little evidence of a decrease in the overall number of T cells in CFS. Nonetheless, some studies report alterations in T cell subsets in CFS patients when compared to healthy controls. For instance, decreases in helper cell populations in conjunction with increases in suppressor and cytotoxic cell markers have been reported in two studies (Klimas *et al.* 1990; Straus *et al.* 1993), while two others have found no differences in these cell populations (Gupta and Vayuvegula 1991; Tirelli *et al.* 1994). Straus *et al.* (1993) also observed a rise in the memory cell population, although this was not confirmed in a more recent study (Peakman *et al.* 1997). The data on NK cells is even more conflicting. Some investigators have shown no differences between CFS patients and controls in the number of NK cells. Others suggest a decrease in numbers, while still others have found an increase in NK cell markers (see Demitrack 1996 for review).

T cell functioning

Investigations of T cell functioning in CFS patients have been somewhat more consistent than the studies on cell counts. CFS patients appear to have depressed NK cell function and reduced lymphocyte production in response to an externally administered stimulant of the immune system (see Vollmer-Conna *et al.* 1998 for review). A more direct test of cellular immune function is to administer antigens under the skin and to measure or observe the reaction of the skin to these antigens. Here the results have been contradictory. One study reported reduced or absent delayed-type hypersensitivity (DTH) skin responses in CFS patients (Lloyd *et al.* 1992), while another found no differences in CFS cases and controls' DTH skin responses to a wide range of antigens (Mawle *et al.* 1997).

Although inconsistencies exist between studies, the chronic immune activation hypothesis has arisen from the results of these studies. This hypothesis suggests that the NK dysfunction or decreases in suppressor T cell populations, reported in a number of studies, result in a persistent hyperimmune response of the remaining cytotoxic cells or T cells which attack altered body cells (Landay *et al.* 1991). This activation may lead to an increase in the production of cellular products such as cytokines, which in turn cause the characteristic symptoms of CFS. This activation hypothesis is the one that is frequently cited by patient journals.

Cytokine abnormalities

Cytokines play a pivotal role in regulating the immune system through stimulating the growth and proliferation of lymphocytes, as well as activating and de-activating the immune processes. Cytokines are thought to produce some of the central nervous system (CNS) symptoms of acute infections such as weakness, fatiguability, hypersomnia and social withdrawal, which play an important part in returning the body to health (Bearn and Wessely 1994). Therefore, citing cytokines as one of the factors in CFS is an attractive hypothesis.

Nevertheless, the only dependable finding is altered in vitro-stimulated cytokine release (Vollmer-Conna *et al.* 1998). In vitro experiments remove cells or cellular products from the body and test their responses to various agents in a laboratory. Thus, they do not necessarily provide an accurate picture of what happens in the body itself. Results from studies of direct measures of circulating cytokines are much less consistent, concluding that levels are either normal, increased or decreased (Demitrack 1996; Vollmer-Conna *et al.* 1998). Lloyd and colleagues (1994) proposed that CFS symptoms are caused by the abnormal release of cytokines in response to exercise, as patients consistently complain that their symptoms are exacerbated by exertion. However, two controlled trials of cytokine production in response to exercise have found no evidence of alteration in cytokine levels in CFS patients (Lloyd *et al.* 1994; Peterson *et al.* 1994).

Clinical implications of the immune findings

The clinical significance of the immunological abnormalities reported is uncertain, for a number of reasons. Most of the abnormalities described do not occur in a number of cases, and differences between CFS patients and controls are not always statistically significant. When compared to classic immunological disorders, the size of the CFS abnormalities is slight and opportunistic infections do not occur. An opportunistic infection is an infection caused by an organism which usually would not cause an illness except in cases where an individual's immune system is compromised. Thus, despite efforts by researchers, it is clear that unlike

HIV-1 infection, or AIDS which is characterised by a distinctive loss of helper T cells, CFS cannot be distinguished by changes in a specific immune cell type alone (Mawle *et al.* 1997).

There is also little evidence to suggest that immune factors are related to severity of symptoms or clinical outcome. Studies which have claimed to show a relationship between severity of symptoms, disability, improvement and immune status have been cross-sectional and fraught with methodological problems (Hassan *et al.* 1998; Landay *et al.* 1991; Masuda *et al.* 1994). As all these studies found an association between severity of CFS and psychiatric status, it is difficult to rule out the possibility that psychological status may be associated with immune findings in CFS. Peakman *et al.* (1997) found no relationship between immune variables and CFS measures of clinical status, except for a weak association between helper T cells and fatigue. However, they found a stronger correlation between measures of depression and T cell counts.

Three longitudinal studies found no correlation between either humoral or cell-mediated immunity and outcome or improvement in CFS (Clark *et al.* 1995; Peakman *et al.* 1997; Wilson *et al.* 1995). Finally, although there have been some reports of successful treatment with immunoregulatory regimes, to date no specific immunoregulatory agent has demonstrated efficacy in repeated, well designed trials (Vollmer-Conna *et al.* 1997; Wilson *et al.* 1994b).

In summary, at this stage the aetiological role of the immune system is uncertain. Studies have been unable to demonstrate a specific relationship between either the clinical symptoms or course of the disorder and immune abnormalities. Why, then, have different immune markers been found in some studies? One possibility is that immune changes are a consequence or a sequel of the condition. Factors such as medication, activity levels, mood and sleep disturbance have all been shown to influence immune factors in healthy controls (Fielding *et al.* 1993; Irwin *et al.* 1994; Kronfol *et al.* 1986). As these factors are commonly altered in CFS patients, it is possible that immune abnormalities arise as a consequence of the disorder. No research to date has addressed this option. Another possibility is that immune disturbances and symptoms of the illness are functionally unrelated, but arise from some other common biological pathway such as the central nervous system (CNS). The anatomical and physiological interrelationship between these two systems lends credence to the idea that immune abnormalities may be secondary to CNS dysfunction.

Central nervous system findings

The popular British and New Zealand patient name for CFS is ME or myalgic encephalomyelitis. When directly translated myalgia means diffuse muscle pain, while encephalomyelitis means an inflammatory condition of the central nervous system. Many of the classic symptoms of CFS such as fatigue, and concentration and memory difficulties could stem from a neurological basis. One CFS patient discloses how even less classic symptoms are attributable to brain dysfunction:

> Let's face it, our nervous systems are jazzed up and very hypersensitive to just about everything. We're sensitive to sound, heat, cold, light, foods, chemicals, emotional upset, and on and on. I wish I could put my brain on 'idle' for a while.

Despite such symptom descriptions and the popularity of the label ME, we have found that few patients in New Zealand actually attribute their CFS to neurological causes (Moss-Morris 1997b). This may be due to the fact that neurological research into CFS is fairly recent and has received less public attention than the viral and immunological theories. Nevertheless, accounts of the role of the CNS are emerging in the self-help literature. A recent self-help journal article by a CFS sufferer explains how emotional symptoms are caused by CNS dysfunction:

> For people with CFS, emotional changes can be just as unsettling as the physical symptoms produced by the illness. Many people do not understand that the emotional roller coaster is as organic as the fever, swollen glands, low blood pressure or any other symptoms of the illness. That is, the illness can produce 'negative emotions' – overwhelming grief, irritability, anxiety, depression and guilt, and these symptoms come and go like all the other symptoms the illness throws at you.
>
> It is thought that the same mechanisms that produce cognitive difficulties – the malfunctioning limbic system and neuroendocrine disturbance – also give rise to changes in emotions. In CFS, neurotransmitter activity is dysregulated on many fronts.
>
> (Booth 1999a:35)

The underlying message of this article is that a person is helpless in the face of his or her brain malfunctioning, even to the point where emotions are uncontrollable. The title of the book *Betrayal by the Brain*, written by Jay Goldstein (1993) on the neurological basis of CFS, embodies this metaphor. Patients' responses on the internet to Jay Goldstein's work were extremely positive. One patient wrote:

> I am so excited about the wonderful article by Dr. Jay Goldstein in the current *CFIDS Chronicle* that I cannot stand it. It all comes together for me that article. I called immediately to get his book that is referenced in the article, but the publishing date has been moved back to June or July. It is a wonderful overview of the neurochemical basis for the brain damage that every doctor with his/her eyes open since Cheney and Petersen have been seeing in CFIDS patients. It draws together the hormonal, neurochemical, and brain damages pieces that I have intuitively felt were there all along, but how to convince anyone when I lose words while I am doing a descriptive analysis. Finally someone without the DD has recognized what many of us have suspected all along.

The CNS hypothesis of CFS suggests that the symptoms of the illness are caused by a dysregulated neuroendocrine system (Demitrack 1993; Demitrack 1996; Goldstein 1993; Jefferies 1994). Dysregulation is thought to occur through a range of stressful events such as viruses, emotional stress, sleep disruption or overwork, which serve to disrupt the integrity of the hypothalamic–pituitary–adrenal (HPA) axis leading to a glucocorticoid deficiency such as decreased levels of cortisol in the body.

The HPA plays a key role in co-ordinating people's physiological response to stress and their cycle of sleeping and waking. The acute stress response is regulated by a complex array of biochemical processes, starting with the release of corticotrophin-releasing hormone (CRH) and arginine vasopressin (AVP) from centres in the brain such as the hypothalamus. These hormones stimulate the release of yet another hormone, adrenocorticotropic hormone (ACTH), from the pituitary gland, which in turn leads to glucocorticoid release from the adrenal gland. Glucocorticoids, such as cortisol, circulating in the blood stream and complex inhibition processes provide negative feedback to the whole system which terminates the HPA activation.

Neuroendocrine studies in chronic fatigue syndrome

There is some evidence of glucocorticoid deficiency in CFS, as some studies have shown decreased cortisol levels in CFS patients when compared to controls (Demitrack *et al.* 1991; MacHale *et al.* 1998; Scott and Dinan 1998; Strickland *et al.* 1998). However, results are not consistent across studies, with some researchers finding no differences in cortisol levels between CFS patients and controls (Bearn *et al.* 1995; Cleare *et al.* 1995; Scott, Medbak and Dinan 1998; Young *et al.* 1998) and one study finding higher levels in CFS patients when compared to controls (Wood *et al.* 1998).

The glucocorticoid deficiency evident in some groups of CFS patients could be caused by a disruption to any part of the HPA system. The most popular theory is that the impairment occurs at or above the level of the hypothalamus. This is based on the finding that CFS patients release less ACTH in response to exogenous hormonal challenges, but have elevated evening ACTH levels in their blood stream (Bearn *et al.* 1995; Demitrack *et al.* 1991; Dinan *et al.* 1997; Scott *et al.* 1998). These exogenous challenges involve administering a manufactured hormonal substance to the subjects that mimics the effects of CRH. These results suggest that impaired activation of CRH could be a likely candidate. There is also some evidence of reduced AVP levels in CFS (Bakheit *et al.* 1993; Demitrack 1993). As both CRH and AVP are produced by the hypothalamus, the results allude to an impairment at the hypothalamic level.

Neurotransmitter function in chronic fatigue syndrome

If the CFS impairment occurs at or above the hypothalamic level, neurotransmitters may play a key role in the dysregulation. Neurotransmitters are bodily chemicals which are responsible for the transmission of nerve impulses across cells. Central neurotransmitters are involved in the regulation of a number of hypothalamic functions. For instance, the neurotransmitter serotonin assists in activating the hypothalamus, while fenfluramine and buspirone stimulate the release of pituitary hormones.

Two of the pituitary hormones stimulated by fenfluramine and buspirone are prolactin and growth hormone. There is some evidence that CFS patients have an increased buspirone-stimulated prolactin release when compared to controls (Bakheit *et al.* 1992; Sharpe *et al.*

1996a). One study also demonstrated a reduced growth hormone response to hypoglycaemia in CFS patients when compared to controls (Allain *et al.* 1997), but this finding is not consistent (Sharpe *et al.* 1996a).

Other studies have investigated prolactin responses to fenfluramine, with mixed results. Two studies were unable to demonstrate any difference between the CFS patients' and controls' prolactin responses to this challenge (Bearn and Wessely 1994; Yatham *et al.* 1995). Nevertheless, a well matched study, comparing both CFS patients without depression and primary depressed patients with controls, demonstrated opposite patterns in the CFS and depressed groups (Cleare *et al.* 1995). Prolactin responses to fenfluramine were lowest in the depressed group and highest in the CFS group. There was a strong negative correlation between the fenfluramine-mediated response and the levels of cortisol in the system, providing further support for a central role in CFS-related hypocortisolism or reduced cortisol levels.

Clinical implications of the HPA findings

Two randomised controlled trials have investigated hydrocortisone treatment for CFS patients in an attempt to ascertain whether increasing cortisol levels can reduce the experience of symptoms (Cleare *et al.* 1999; McKenzie *et al.* 1998). Both trials showed some benefits for the hydrocortisone groups but there was no long-term follow-up to determine whether the improvement would be sustained. There were also a number of negative side-effects suggesting that hydrocortisone may not be a viable option for treatment. Nevertheless, these studies do suggest that reduced cortisol levels may contribute in some way to CFS symptoms.

Less certain is what causes the cortisol changes in the first place. As we have seen, most of the research in this area assumes it comes from a primary CNS deficit. It is also a possibility that the alterations in the HPA are a consequence of an ongoing chronic condition rather than a causal factor. There is evidence that both emotional and behavioural factors can cause similar neuroendocrine disruption. A recent study on healthy controls showed that perceived stress was associated with lower cortisol secretion (Pruessner, Helhammer and Kirschbaum 1999). An investigation on a small sample of nurses after they had completed five days of night-shift work found that they demonstrated changes to cortisol and ACTH levels that were similar to those reported in CFS patients (Leese *et al.* 1996). Many CFS patients have an erratic sleep pattern as they tend to nap during the day if they are tired and then have difficulties sleeping at night. CFS patients also tend to lead sedentary lives and when compared to healthy controls they are significantly less physically fit (McCully, Sisto and Natelson 1996b). Consequently, neuroendocrine findings in CFS may reflect a disruption to the sleep–wake cycle, or reductions in physical activity.

Support for this idea comes from a study which showed that CFS patients have a disrupted circadian rhythm (Williams *et al.* 1996). Circadian rhythms are our natural 24-hour biological cycles which help to control our patterns of sleep and alertness. Things like international air travel and poor sleep habits can disturb these natural rhythms. The symptoms of disturbed circadian rhythms are similar to the cardinal symptoms of CFS, namely tiredness, impaired concentration, and intellectual impairment. Thus, CFS patients' disrupted daily routines may result in a feeling of constant jet lag which is reflected in subtle alteration to the HPA.

Neuroimaging studies

Scanning techniques that investigate both the anatomical structure and the functioning of the brain have been used in CFS studies. Studies investigating structural abnormalities in CFS patients have largely utilised magnetic resonance imaging (MRI). This is a highly sophisticated technique which employs magnetic fields, radio waves and computerised enhancement to map out brain structure. MRI studies have reported a variety of changes in the white matter of the brain in a greater percentage of CFS patients when compared to controls (Buchwald *et al.* 1992; Natelson *et al.* 1993, Schwartz 1994). However, the differences have not always been significant and MRI abnormalities have not resolved with clinical improvement (Schwartz *et al.* 1994a). The only CFS study to include depressed patients as control subjects found no significant group differences, with white matter brain lesions being correlated with current intellectual under-functioning (Cope *et al.* 1995). Consequently, to date, there is no MRI abnormality that is characteristic of CFS patients and any observed abnormalities may reflect alterations in attention and concentration.

Functional neuroimaging looks at the actual activity within the brain. These studies have utilised single-photon-emission-computed tomographic scanning (SPECT) to measure cerebral blood flow. In SPECT radioactively tagged chemicals are introduced into the brain. These serve as markers of blood flow in the different regions of the brain which can be monitored with X-rays. While this technique can be used to investigate blood flow during different activities, in the CFS studies it has largely been employed to investigate resting regional blood flow. A range of abnormalities has been reported in CFS patients, although no definite pattern has emerged (see Cope and David 1996 for review). SPECT studies, which have included patients with major depression as a comparison group, report mixed results. Two studies were unable to demonstrate substantial differences between CFS and depression (Goldstein *et al.* 1995; Schwartz *et al.* 1994b). Another reported that while both the depressed and CFS groups showed altered blood flow patterns, the alterations in each of the groups were in different regions of the brain (Fischler *et al.* 1996).

Clinical implications of the neuroimaging studies

Few studies have investigated clinical features of CFS in relation to SPECT abnormalities. Scharwtz *et al.* (1994a) reported that improvement in CFS over a six-month period was associated with blood flow deficits, but they only studied four patients. Fischler *et al.* (1996) found positive correlations between higher frontal blood flow and depression ratings, cognitive complaints and self-reported physical impairment. However, as frontal blood flow did not distinguish between CFS patients and healthy controls in this study, these results are difficult to interpret. Finally, as a feeling of extreme tiredness and weakness following exercise is a chief complaint of CFS patients, Peterson *et al.* (1994) investigated whether exercise affected cerebral blood flow in CFS. They were unable to demonstrate a significant difference between patients and controls. In conclusion, while imaging studies provide some support for the hypothesis that CNS disturbance is more evident in patients than controls, the profound lack of information regarding the clinical significance of neuroimaging abnormalities, together with varied results and overlap with depression, makes it unlikely that brain abnormalities hold the answer for many CFS patients.

Neuropsychological studies

Another way in which investigators have tried to quantify CNS involvement in CFS is through the use of standardised laboratory tests of neuropsychological functioning. These tests measure intellectual ability, memory and attentional functions and the speed with which an individual processes information. While mild impairments have been documented, particularly on tasks demanding a high speed of information processing and complex attentional processes, there is no evidence that these impairments are indicative of an organic brain disorder (see Moss-Morris *et al.* 1996a; Wearden and Appleby 1996 for reviews). Deficits when they are reported are traditionally within one standard deviation from the norm. There is also some evidence that neuropsychological impairments are associated with mood, sleep disturbance and symptom reports in CFS suggesting that these cognitive impairments may be secondary features to other aspects of the disorder.

Sleep abnormalities

The presence of disrupted circadian rhythms, coupled with the fact that sleep disturbance is one of the key symptoms described by CFS sufferers, has led some investigators to suggest that CFS may represent a primary sleep disorder. Cytokines and serotonin also have sleep-promoting properties, so the CFS findings in these areas could reflect a primary sleep problem.

Polysomnographic studies, which measure brain waves during sleep, have documented a somewhat inconsistent range of abnormalities in CFS samples. There are two types of sleep, non-REM sleep and REM sleep. REM stands for rapid eye movements, so during REM sleep these eye movements occur, while in non-REM sleep they do not. Non-REM sleep is further divided into four stages of sleep and each of these stages has characteristic brain waves associated with it. People who report symptoms of chronic tiredness, unrefreshing sleep and musculoskeletal discomfort have demonstrated prominent alpha intrusions in their brain waves during non-REM sleep (Macfarlane *et al.* 1996). Alpha waves usually occur in drowsy stages just before one falls asleep. This abnormality is referred to as alpha-delta sleep. One study reported alpha-delta sleep in a small sample of CFS patients (Whelton, Salit and Moldofsky 1992), although a later study did not (Manu *et al.* 1994). Zubieta *et al.* (1993) found that CFS patients spent an increased amount of time in stage four and in delta sleep, when compared to both healthy controls and depressed patients. However, these alterations in sleep patterns have not been replicated in other CFS studies (Morriss *et al.* 1993), one of which even reported a lower percentage of stage four sleep in CFS patients (Fischler *et al.* 1997c). Finally, significantly lower levels of REM sleep have been reported in some studies (Stores, Fry and Crawford 1998; Whelton *et al.* 1992) but not others (Fischler *et al.* 1997c; Morriss *et al.* 1993).

A more consistent finding is that CFS patients have higher levels of disruptions to their sleep during the night and significantly less sleep efficiency (Fischler *et al.* 1997c; Stores *et al.* 1998; Whelton *et al.* 1992). These sleep abnormalities do not seem to be related to either the presence of co-occurring psychiatric disorder, mood disturbance or disability in CFS (Fischler *et al.* 1997c). Further investigations are needed to determine whether these sleep difficulties account for the unrefreshing sleep which is a defining symptom of the disorder. A CFS patient, Theresa, provides a graphic account of the sensation of unrefreshing sleep:

> I would wake and feel as if I had run a hundred miles. I was too tired and achey to get out of bed to make a cup of tea. On one of these days I should have been on a cycle outing from London to Brighton. I lay in bed feeling I'd ridden the course several times over.
>
> (Theresa cited in Steincamp 1989:34)

The cause of this sleep disturbance is still unclear, as there does not appear to be a consistent abnormality in sleep architecture that distinguishes CFS patients as a group. Nevertheless, the results from sleep studies are enthusiastically reported in patient journals as evidence of the organic nature of the condition. A recent self-help journal reports:

> The awful disturbed sleep that has been Moldofsky's research interest for years – is truly that. He showed all sorts of 'stuff ups' ... All these disrupted hormones add up to sleep that doesn't do what it should for us. The phase shift of cortisol is advanced by about 45 mins and likely why we can be up late at night, but can't wake up till late morning. All the abnormalities can account for the arousal disturbance we get throughout the night. In other words our circadian rhythm is corrupted!
>
> (Booth 1999b:17)

While the HPA alterations may indeed account for some of the sleep disturbances, another possibility not mentioned in our local self-help journal is that behavioural patterns of sleep may also be a factor. Many CFS patients report that they need to sleep during the day. Daytime sleep may result in less efficient and more disturbed night-time patterns. In addition, as we will see in the next section, CFS patients show evidence of deconditioning or extreme loss of fitness due to lack of activity. These factors may also contribute to sleep problems.

Muscle, cardiovascular and respiratory abnormalities

Another characteristic symptom of CFS is the experience of extreme post-exertional malaise. Patients frequently relate that while they can tolerate physical exertion reasonably well, six to twenty-four hours later they experience marked worsening of their symptoms, particularly pain and weakness in the muscles (Komaroff and Buchwald 1991).

We asked 282 CFS patients what would happen to them if they exerted themselves (Petrie *et al.* 1995). Almost all patients felt that this would have a negative impact on their symptoms. Here are two typical examples of the responses:

> I would be even worse off. All symptoms aggravated. Severe muscle and joint pain. Painful to move or touch. Chronic depression would return (the depression comes after, not before, the physical symptoms). The slightest movement is painful – all over. I'd be back to sleeping all day and night.

> Extreme physical and mental fatigue requiring several days of complete rest before able to start on light activities again. Extremely unwell feelings. Risk of flu, chest pain, abdominal cramps, muscle fatigue at a gross level, memory loss, lower limb weakness.

These patient reports have led to the suggestion that abnormalities of muscle or the cardiovascular system, or both, may be the major site of dysfunction in CFS. Researchers have therefore investigated the tissues and cells of patients' muscles, as well as their physiological responses to physically demanding situations.

Muscle histopathology

Minor abnormalities of the cells of the muscle have been documented using a range of laboratory techniques such as a reduction in the breakdown or uptake of oxygen by the muscles (see McCully *et al.* 1996b for review). However, these small abnormalities have no demonstrable clinical significance and the findings have not been replicated in all studies. In all likelihood these minor abnormalities reflect deconditioning effects. Inactivity has been shown to have negative effects on the way in which muscles metabolise or break down oxygen, and CFS patients report significantly reduced activity levels together with frequent periods of bedrest (McCully *et al.* 1996b).

Exercise performance and muscle functioning

The deconditioning hypothesis has been supported by a number of laboratory exercise studies which have found that CFS patients have a reduced exercise capacity when compared to healthy controls, as well as significantly reduced oxygen uptake and lactate levels during recovery (De Lorenzo *et al.* 1998; Edwards *et al.* 1993; Fischler *et al.* 1997b; Sisto *et al.* 1996). Muscles break down or metabolise oxygen as an energy source. One of the by-products of this process is lactate. These findings were against the background of essentially normal heart and lung functioning.

Investigations of muscle functioning have documented normal muscle strength, endurance and recovery in CFS patients, substantiating the view that the muscle is unlikely to be the major site of dysfunction in CFS (see McCully *et al.* 1996b for review). One other possibility is that the nerves which feed or enervate muscle tissue are affected in CFS, as the muscle weakness in neurological disorders such as MS is related to nerve involvement. However, a study comparing MS and CFS patients found that only the MS group demonstrated objective signs of muscle fatigue, which were correlated with their other symptoms of nerve involvement (Djaldetti *et al.* 1996).

Perhaps the most striking finding is that although, as we have seen at the beginning of this section, CFS patients complain that symptoms get much worse after even mild exertion, this complaint has not been substantiated. Two studies conducted a 24-hour follow-up of CFS patients after they had completed a bout of exhaustive exercise. There was no evidence of alterations to muscle metabolism (McCully *et al.* Leigh 1996a) and patients reported a decrease rather than an increase in symptoms (Lloyd *et al.* 1994). A longer-term study reported a reduction in activity levels following exercise, but this occurred almost two weeks after the exercise and was substantially less than the self-reports suggest (Sisto *et al.* 1998).

Overall, findings from objective laboratory studies on muscle structure and functioning are in stark contrast to the degree of patients' complaints. There is no evidence that exercise has detrimental effects on symptoms and in fact it may even be helpful. The deconditioning findings confirm that decreased activity needs to be investigated in the light of other organic findings.

Hypotension

A group of investigators from the Johns Hopkins Center in Baltimore have conducted two studies which they claim support the hypothesis that CFS is related to neurally mediated hypotension (Bou-Holaigah *et al.* 1995; Rowe *et al.* 1995). Neurally mediated hypotension is a disorder of low blood pressure related to the functioning of one part of the nervous system, the autonomic nervous system. The autonomic nervous system regulates the body's vital functions including the activity of the heart and cardiac system. The symptoms of neurally mediated hypotension are severe light-headedness or a brief lapse in consciousness when altering bodily posture. One way this is assessed is by placing patients on a tilted table for extended periods of time. The Johns Hopkins group reported that 95 per cent of CFS patients demonstrated an abnormal tilt table test result compared to 29 per cent of healthy controls (Bou-Holaigah *et al.* 1995; Rowe *et al.* 1995). Forty per cent of the patients with abnormal responses reported partial or total resolution of their CFS symptoms following drug therapy directed at neurally mediated hypotension (Bou-Holaigah *et al.* 1995). However, as the trial did not include a placebo control, and 30–50 per cent of CFS patients demonstrate improvement in the placebo arms of controlled trials, these results may well reflect nothing more than the placebo effect. A later study conducted by another group found that only 25 per cent of their CFS sample showed tilt table abnormalities (Freeman and Komaroff 1997). Further, longitudinal and population-based studies have demonstrated an association between both depression and inactivity, and low blood pressure (Wessely 1995c). Neither of these factors was controlled for in these studies. Clearly, the claims made by these investigators are far more conclusive than their methodology warrants.

However, as with a number of other organic findings, the results are eagerly picked up by CFS sufferers. The self-help journals contain numerous reports from patients of how they have increased their daily salt intake with positive results in response to the Johns Hopkins studies. A general practitioner weekly magazine published a dramatic account of a patient's experience at the Johns Hopkins Center entitled 'Tilting table creates CFS horror and hope' (Crashley 1997). This patient, Sandra Crashley, a president of an ME support service, vividly describes the symptoms she experienced while on the tilt table:

> Other common symptoms of ME/CFS surfaced in intensity during the 45 minutes such as sore eyes and sensations of burning eyeballs which blurred my vision; dry mouth and throat; panic feelings of being unable to breathe … excruciating pain in the back of the neck; buzzing in the ears; my hearing intensified as I lost the ability to sift out unwanted noises; thick cloggy, foggy brain; creepy crawly feelings of insecurity …
>
> (Crashley 1997:36)

She goes on to explain to the general practitioners that Dr Rowe is advising patients to increase their salt intake to 2–3 teaspoons a day and their water intake to 2 litres per day. She is hoping to raise research funding so that a trial can be conducted on fludrocortisone medication for this disorder.

Respiratory abnormalities

Hyperventilation or over-breathing is yet another posited cause for CFS. Based on patients' perceptions of their feelings of shortness of breath following voluntary hyperventilation, Rosen and colleagues (Rosen *et al.* 1990) concluded that CFS was nothing more than chronic hyperventilation. Subsequent studies using more rigorous methods to measure hyperventilation, such as measuring decreased levels of carbon dioxide in the system, have shown that carbon dioxide levels cannot account for either the degree of symptoms nor functional impairment reported by CFS patients (Lavietes *et al.* 1996; Saisch *et al.* 1994). CFS patients with and without hyperventilation report the same severity of fatigue-related symptoms (Bazelmans *et al.* 1997). Saisch *et al.* (1994) also found that CFS patients with unequivocal hyperventilation had either panic disorder or asthma which would account for the decreased levels of carbon dioxide in their system. Consequently, while hyperventilation may contribute to the experience of symptoms in some CFS cases, it is extremely unlikely that it is the sole cause of the debilitating illness.

Allergy, diets and pollutants

After viruses and immune dysfunction, allergens and pollutants are CFS patients' most favoured attributions (Moss-Morris 1997b). Claims that a wide variety of sensitivities are major causes of the illness, together with diets and strategies to combat these problems, pervade the CFS self-help literature. Sherry Rodgers, a general practitioner, describes the beginnings of her chemical sensitivity and ongoing fatigue in a local ME journal.

> I was normal until six years ago I was at the bank and went on my coffee break. When I returned I began getting sick. I noticed my chair was wet, and I learned that the exterminator had just been through for his routine spraying of insecticide. Over the next hour I starting feeling really sick. They told me to go home, that my symptoms would wear off. But each time I tried to return in the next few weeks, I felt so sick I couldn't stay.
>
> (Rodgers 1992:26)

A commonly held patient belief is that allergens cause CFS symptoms through their effect on the immune system. This is seen to create a vicious cycle, with the compromised immune system causing increased sensitivities to a wider range of substances. For instance, Rosalie, a long-term CFS sufferer, believes that an initial sensitivity to natural gas triggered her ongoing problems:

> We removed all the gas from the house (very expensive) and I left my job because by this time I was unable to function with gas and it was hoped that by taking these measures, my immune system should settle down and that I should improve. But 5 yrs [sic] later I am as sensitive to gas (and a multitude of things) as ever ... If I ignore my restraints and go into an environment of smoke, perfume, and alcohol, I know that not only would my immediate problem be intense pain, weakness and wheezing but also my immune system would be so stirred up that for weeks afterwards I would be overreacting to every allergen I came into contact with and almost every food which at present I can just tolerate sparingly, would be poison to me.
>
> (cited in Horne 1992:4–5)

This concept of allergens and pollutants has been particularly popular in New Zealand where a number of CFS patients have had chemical toxicity diagnosed by a technique known as electro-acupuncture, but there have been no objective studies published which allow evaluation of this technique (Murdoch 1988). A study which measured levels of lead, mercury and arsenic, all of which are associated with fatigue, found no evidence of accumulation of these elements in CFS patients (Mawle *et al.* 1997).

There is some objective evidence of greater sensitivity to allergens in CFS patients. Three studies reported that 50–77 per cent of CFS subjects demonstrate positive skin tests to a variety of allergens (Conti *et al.* 1996; Straus *et al.* 1988b). However, Mawle *et al.* (1997) found no laboratory evidence for the increased incidence of allergies in CFS patients, despite the fact that they reported more allergy-associated symptoms than did controls. Other studies have also found little association between reports of allergies in CFS and objective evidence of these allergies (Conti *et al.* 1996; Steinberg *et al.* 1996). A randomised controlled trial of the antihistamine Terfenadine showed no treatment effect for CFS patients, either with or without allergies (Steinberg *et al.* 1996).

Food intolerances together with chronic candidiasis has been a particularly popular CFS attribution. Candidiasis is an infection caused by a yeast-like fungus which can affect the gut and other internal organs. Sylvia Horne, a CFS sufferer, describes the problem of chronic candidiasis as follows:

> Yeast allergy is one of the most universally common – a fungus parasite of the gut normally kept in check by the immune system, but it can become systemic, or cause a skin infection. It causes leaky gut mucosa, letting toxic substances into the body and causes immunosupression and increased production of corticosterone. It causes many symptoms like ME and allergy – food cravings, feeling bad all over, hypoglycaemia, chemical sensitivities.
>
> (Horne 1992:67)

Judith Lopez, in an article entitled 'What's eating you', describes her long-term battle with CFS and how a nutritionist finally diagnosed her problem as candidiasis:

> She also told me I had all the symptoms of Candidiasis, or yeast infestation, and gave me an antifungal herb called Paramycocidin ... Something *had* in fact been 'eating me' all those years, a strange growth-like monster from a science-fiction story. It had established

itself in my intestinal tract and was poisoning me with its metabolic by-products and destroying my immune system.

(Lopez 1991:12)

To date, none of the diets promoted for the relief of CFS symptoms and to combat candida has been substantiated by clinical research (Morris and Stare 1993). Some studies have made remarkable claims for the effectiveness of dietary supplements in CFS, but these results have not been replicated in subsequent randomised trials (see Wessely, Hotopf and Sharpe 1998 for review). Further, reports of food intolerance are not always substantiated by objective data. In a study of patients with chronic fatigue, no laboratory differences were found between patients who did and did not report food intolerance (Manu, Matthews and Lane 1993b). Rather, food allergies were positively associated with a general tendency to report physical complaints. Evidence of psychological disorder or distress has also been related to unsubstantiated food allergies in the general population (Parker *et al.* 1991). Consequently, the lack of consistency between symptoms and objective evidence of allergies makes the aetiological role of allergens uncertain.

The latest 'diagnostic' test

Despite the wide range of organic factors studied, researchers have been unable to find a definitive diagnostic test for CFS. There is little evidence at this stage that physiological variables correlate with symptoms and disability in CFS. The exception is two recent reports from an Australian group of researchers who claim they have devised an objective test for CFS which confirms the molecular basis of the disorder (McGregor *et al.* 1996a; McGregor *et al.* 1996b). In a study of twenty patients they demonstrated that CFS subjects had alterations in their urinary metabolites when compared to healthy controls. Urinary metabolites are the by-products or substances found in urine and produced by the metabolic action of the body. Two of these metabolites correlated highly with the symptoms of the disorder. The authors believed their findings were suggestive of alterations in metabolism and the body's ability to regulate itself and concluded that their study 'provided strong evidence for an etiological association between these metabolites and CFS' (McGregor *et al.* 1996a:7). It is obvious from a scientific point of view that aetiological conclusions cannot be drawn from a single correlational study conducted on a small sample. No attempt has been made to control for possible confounding factors, such as inactivity or sleep disturbance, both of which can alter metabolism. Further, the correlations between the urinary metabolites and some of the measures of psychopathology reported in the results section, are not mentioned in the discussion as having any clinical significance. While urinary metabolites may prove to be a useful indicator of illness severity, substantial work is needed before any aetiological conclusions can be drawn.

Despite the preliminary nature of the research a recent letter from the editor in a self-help journal states:

> In mid-August I took the Newcastle research urine test … and am eagerly awaiting the results … The day after doing the test I began the Johns Hopkins protocol for treating Neurally Mediated Hypotension … and again I'll keep you posted.
>
> (Booth 1996:2).

As discussed earlier, the Johns Hopkins study of neurally mediated hypotension was an uncontrolled trial conducted on a small sample of CFS patients. Similar responses have been made to the earlier claims, and at different points in time patients may have been eagerly awaiting results from viral antibody titres, hyperventilation tests, or maybe NK cell counts. Clearly, the need to have a legitimate marker for the illness is paramount for CFS patients.

Summary and conclusions

This chapter illustrates that a large amount of research has been conducted in the past decade in an attempt to substantiate the physical nature of CFS. Negative or conflicting findings in one area have resulted in research shifting its focus to a different bodily system. Initial investigations focused on the role of viruses, but no single pathogen was associated with the condition. Prospective studies suggest that while most cases are not caused by a virus, a small minority are triggered by severe viral infections, such as glandular fever and hepatitis. These results led some investigators to propose that CFS represents an immune-related disorder, which can be triggered by any number of viruses. However, studies of the immune system have been unable to demonstrate a consistent immunological deficit in CFS. While some patients do demonstrate a mild form of non-specific immune activation or altered functioning of certain cells of the immune system, or both, there does not appear to be a relationship between clinical symptoms of the disorder and immune abnormalities.

The possibility that the immune alterations are secondary to a more central dysfunction led to the formation of new hypotheses about the involvement of the CNS. There is some evidence that CFS patients may have a mild form of hypocortisolism which is associated with a centrally mediated increase in serotonin function. Neuroimaging studies have also found evidence for altered cerebral blood flow in CFS patients, while sleep studies suggest alterations in sleep patterns. However, there is great variability between studies and no distinct abnormality seems to distinguish CFS patients. A disrupted HPA axis seems to be the most plausible hypothesis at this stage as it could account for altered sleep patterns as well as changes in the immune system. However, as neuroendocrine changes similar to those found in CFS patients have been associated with both shift work and stress levels in healthy people, it is possible that the HPA disturbances are a result, rather than a cause of the illness. Similarly, although some studies have documented evidence of hypotension and changes in muscle histology in CFS patients, these could be the result of inactivity. Hyperventilation has also been a suspect, but it is more than likely a secondary feature of panic disorder or asthma.

Thus, the causal role of physical factors in CFS has yet to be determined, as has the clinical significance of the physiological abnormalities. Longitudinal studies have been unable to document a relationship between ongoing disability in CFS and physiological abnormalities. Despite the lack of prospective evidence for organic factors in CFS, it is not uncommon for claims of causation to be made from preliminary, uncontrolled results from new areas of investigation. Patients, desperate for people to acknowledge their suffering and disability, follow the results of these studies closely and are quick to try any new remedies or undergo any new tests which may objectively confirm their illness. While there are sufficient physiological changes to suggest that biological factors do play a role in CFS, the apparent discrepancy between objective results and subjective symptom reports leaves little doubt that factors other than organic abnormalities must be contributing to the debilitating nature of CFS.

Chapter 4

Psychiatric illness and the social context of chronic fatigue syndrome

Many of the organic hypotheses arose from the observation that CFS shares a number of symptoms with certain medical conditions. However, it could be argued that there is even greater symptom overlap with primary psychiatric disorder. Debilitating fatigue and sleep disturbances are consistently associated with psychiatric disorder in studies of the community, primary care and tertiary care (David *et al.* 1990; Pawlikowska *et al.* 1994). Up to 85 per cent of CFS patients report depression as a key symptom, while between 50 and 70 per cent report anxiety (Komaroff and Buchwald 1991). Further, the current definitions of CFS are based on descriptive phenomenology, the traditional domain of psychiatric, rather than medical, diagnoses.

In the first part of this chapter we review the evidence for overlap between CFS and psychiatric illness and outline a range of hypotheses which have been put forward to explain the findings. Typical examples of patients' responses to these psychological findings are also presented. The last part of this chapter is devoted to understanding the social factors which contribute to patients' attitudes towards psychiatry. How these social factors influence CFS patients' experiences of the medical profession and their pathways through diagnosis is also discussed. Finally, an integrated model of CFS which incorporates the biological, psychological and social aspects of the illness is presented.

Chronic fatigue syndrome and diagnosed psychiatric disorder

At least seventeen published studies have attempted to ascertain the incidence of psychiatric disorder in CFS, using a variety of standardised diagnostic interviews (see Abbey 1996 for review). The weight of evidence suggests that CFS patients have a higher incidence of both life-time and current psychiatric disorders when compared to healthy controls, other medically ill patients, and population norms. On average around 60 to 70 per cent of patients meet criteria for a comorbid psychiatric condition, although figures as high as 86 per cent have been quoted (Katon *et al.* 1991) and as low as 24.5 per cent (Hickie *et al.* 1990).

The most convincing evidence for the role of psychiatric disorder in CFS comes from two prospective cohort studies of patients attending primary care (Cope *et al.* 1996; Wessely *et al.* 1996a). New cases of CFS were associated with previously recorded psychiatric diagnoses and prescriptions of psychotropic medication at a substantially higher rate than matched non-fatigued controls. In line with the majority of retro-spective studies, between two-thirds and three-quarters of the patients with CFS had a concurrent psychiatric disorder, even when excluding fatigue as a diagnostic criterion, compared to less than a quarter of controls.

Although there are a handful of exceptions, the results of studies investigating the incidence of psychiatric disorder in CFS have been remarkably consistent. Yet, patient journals and self-help pamphlets either avoid reporting the findings from these studies or typically respond as follows:

> Anybody producing a paper of just about any degree of mediocrity linking ME/CF(ID)S with psychological causes and theories will have no trouble getting it published. No matter that these papers might be riddled with logical errors and simple ignorance. That such bad papers are ever written is a great pity with potentially tragic consequences: several ANZMES members wrote to us in distress to tell of the damage done to their credibility among family and friends.
>
> (*Meeting-Place* 1990:31)

Not only do the methods of these studies come under attack, but the researchers themselves may be personally denigrated. A CFIDS chat group member writes:

> Wow! With 'research' help like this, from those omnipotent experts (the Shrinks), should there be any wonder at all that cheap-opportunists like the media so often jump at the chance to 'psychologize' and 'satirize' our CFS illness? In a world of 'diminishing scapegoats,' CFSers are a valuable commodity, if for no other reason than that we

fulfill the need for public buffoon figures, thanks to this sort of 'bad press.' I'm curious: Was this JPR article author a Canadian or Briton; or merely European? (Not that I have anything against any of those groups …) I only ask this because I'm wondering WHERE on the planet this type of 'thinking' passes for 'research'; and the spelling looks rather British. His Freudian 'take' on the situation is certainly revealing, nauseating, and passe to the nth …

Despite these protestations, depressive disorders are commonly diagnosed among CFS patients, followed by anxiety disorders and somatisation disorder: a chronic psychiatric condition characterised by multiple physical complaints. While some studies have also reported the presence of hypochondriasis, conversion disorder, substance abuse and eating disorders, the number of patients meeting criteria for these disorders is minimal. In fact, both substance abuse and eating disorders are exclusion criteria in the latest CDC definition of CFS (Fukuda *et al.* 1994).

Chronic fatigue syndrome and depression

Around two-thirds of CFS patients would have met criteria for a diagnosis of depression at some stage in their life, even when controlling for overlapping symptoms such as fatigue (Bombardier and Buchwald 1995; Clark *et al.* 1995; Katon *et al.* 1991; Wessely *et al.* 1996a; Wood *et al.* 1991). Major depression is the most common diagnosis, with around 25 per cent of patients meeting criteria for dysthymia or low mood over a long period of time. A number of hypotheses have been proposed to explain the overlap between depression and CFS. These include the possibilities that CFS is an atypical form of depression, depression is a risk factor for the development of CFS, depression is a result of having a chronic physical illness, or CFS and depression arise from a common underlying mechanism (Abbey and Garfinkel 1991; Ray 1991). Each of these hypotheses is considered in turn.

Chronic fatigue syndrome as a form of depression

In some of the formative work in the area, Manu and colleagues (1988; 1993a) proposed that the overlap in the diagnosis and symptoms of the two disorders meant that CFS was either misdiagnosed depression or an atypical form of depression. However, studies which have taken a closer look at the two conditions reveal some important differences. CFS patients consistently report lower mean scores on depression inventories than do primary depressed patients, although their scores are within the depressed range (Hickie *et al.* 1990; Johnson, DeLuca and Natelson 1996a; Moss-Morris 1997; Wessely and Powell 1989). Higher scores for depressed patients are largely accounted for by self-reproach symptoms, such as guilt, low self-esteem and suicidal ideation (Johnson, DeLuca and Natelson 1996a; Moss-Morris 1997; Wessely and Powell 1989). Similarly, the classic cognitive style evident in depressed patients where they tend to make internal attributions for negative interpersonal happenings is not evident in CFS patients. CFS patients do, however, report higher levels of somatic symptoms than patients with depression (Johnson, DeLuca and Natelson 1996a; Moss-Morris and Petrie 1997). The qualitative differences between CFS and depression are often substantiated by patient reports. One patient explains:

> I've had depression before, sort of not very badly, but I have been depressed enough to sort of you know, to be sent to a psychiatrist and put on antidepressants ... And for me it is nothing like that. It was very clearly a physical disability ... I could say definitely I wasn't depressed. I got miserable at times because it is miserable being in that situation.
>
> (cited in Ax *et al.* 1997:251)

Clinical observations also suggest another key difference. Unlike depressed patients who characteristically report a loss of interest in daily activities, CFS patients express frustration at their inability to do things (Surawy *et al.* 1995). This feeling was typified by one of our CFS research participants:

> One of the aspects of the illness not often mentioned is the feelings of frustration it causes. Even after greatly reducing my expectations, the gap between all the things I want to do and the small amount I can do is so vast. Another is the difficulty making plans. All plans must be capable of being unmade on the day if I am too tired or sleepy.

Not only are there phenomenological differences, but there also appear to be physiological differences between CFS and depression. Neuro-endocrine studies have shown that CFS patients and depressed patients have opposing patterns of responses to neurotransmitter challenges. While depression appears to be associated with higher levels of cortisol, CFS is associated with lower levels of the same hormone (Cleare *et al.* 1995). There is also some evidence of different sleep disturbances in these two groups (Zubieta *et al.* 1993). The most recent finding is that prolonged fatigue and psychological distress may be determined in part by independent genetic and environmental factors (Hickie *et al.* 1999).

Further evidence for the difference between CFS and depression comes from preliminary treatment trials of antidepressant medications. Two randomised, double-blind, placebo-controlled trials of antidepressant medication failed to show improvement in CFS patients (Natelson *et al.* 1996; Vercoulen *et al.* 1996a). While another trial did find a short-term antidepressant effect for Fluoxetine in CFS patients, the drug had no effect on their levels of disability or fatigue (Wearden *et al.* 1998). Taken together, the weight of evidence argues against CFS as a form of depression.

Depression as a risk factor for chronic fatigue syndrome

Thus, the research on CFS and depression has largely established two facts: there is a high incidence of lifetime depressive disorder in CFS, and there are subtle differences in the symptom profiles and physiology of patients with primary depression and those with CFS. However, these facts tell us little about the aetiology of the condition. The fact that depression predates the onset of CFS in the majority of cases and the high incidence of lifetime depressive disorder suggests an aetiological role. However, just how depression leads to CFS is uncertain.

Three prospective studies of the role of viruses in CFS found that psychiatric disorder and psychological distress at or before clinical presentation predicted the development of post-viral fatigue six to twenty-four months after infection (Cope *et al.* 1994; Hotopf, Noah and Wessely 1996; Wessely *et al.* 1995b). However, other factors such as fatigue at presentation, prolonged bed rest, time off work and symptom attributional style were also associated with ongoing fatigue (Cope *et al.* 1994; Hotopf, Noah and Wessely 1996). When these variables were entered into a regression equation together with psychological morbidity, a psychiatric history was no longer a significant predictor of CFS (Cope *et al.* 1994). The only significant predictor of a psychiatric diagnosis post-virally was past psychiatric history. As such, premorbid psychiatric disorder may be a more important risk factor for Chronic Fatigue with comorbid depression rather than CFS *per se.*

These results suggest that while depression may be a risk factor for CFS it is unlikely to be a sole cause of the illness. Depression may act as a risk factor for CFS through prolonged convalescence leading to physical deconditioning, which in itself causes symptoms of fatigue. In addition, psychological morbidity may also create some of the symptoms directly due to the overlap between CFS and psychiatric disorder. Alternatively, depression may act as a risk factor, by altering CNS or immune system functioning, or both, which in turn may cause ongoing symptoms (Demitrack 1996).

Depression as a reaction to chronic fatigue syndrome

Another possibility is that depression in CFS is a normal reaction to a debilitating organic condition. Proponents of this position point out that on average one-third of patients do not meet criteria for any psychiatric disorder, and those that do are phenomenologically different from people with a primary psychiatric disturbance (Hickie *et al.* 1990; Johnson, DeLuca and Natelson 1996a). Further, debilitating physical illness is an established risk factor for the development of depression.

This explanation is favoured by the patients themselves. A recent support group information sheet for CFS sufferers states that 'most importantly, the depression seen in patients with ME is "reactive" or secondary to the stress of severe persisting symptoms'. In line with this thinking, David Thompson, a CFS sufferer, explains in an article written for *Mental Health News* the importance of seeing depression as a reaction rather than a diagnosis:

> ... ME represents a syndrome of various organic causes; it is no more psychological than any other chronic disease. Although it has mercifully not happened to me, I know many patients who have had to argue their way out of an all too vague psychological diagnosis before less understood physical entities, especially tentative 'ME', can even be considered. This burden of proof is very stressful. We are already struggling just to think straight, to understand what is happening to us and to cope ... Emotional and cognitive problems result directly from the disease, but also from the disintegration of a healthy life. There is a traumatic assault on self-hood as we lose things by which we defined ourselves: relationships, careers, study, leisure.
>
> (Thompson 1992:26)

Similarly, a CFS participant in a recent study of ours explained that doctors' reactions were one of the most disturbing aspects of the illness and that this in itself could lead to depression. He explains:

> Disturbing aspects such as lack of believability from doctors, ignorance, e.g. depression is caused by ME they think it is ME ... Because it is not 'recognised' by many doctors patients are labelled neurotic, hysterical etc. even in the face of abnormal test results. This all leads to depression and some to suicide.

While depression may well be a reaction to CFS in some cases, it is unlikely to be the sole explanation for the overlap between the disorders. Studies which have compared CFS to a range of other medical illnesses, including rheumatoid arthritis, MS, neuromuscular disorders and myopathies have consistently reported significantly higher levels of depression in CFS (Johnson, DeLuca and Natelson 1996a; Katon *et al.* 1991; Pepper *et al.* 1993; Wessely and Powell 1989; Wood *et al.* 1991). The fact that CFS patients also have a higher incidence of premorbid depression compared to these groups confirms that their psychological distress is not just a reaction to physical morbidity.

Depression and chronic fatigue syndrome as features of the same underlying condition

If depression is neither a result nor a cause of CFS, another alternative is that these two disorders arise from a common underlying pathological mechanism. This hypothesis is based on the notion that the underlying mechanism is biological and more than likely involves the CNS (Abbey and Garfinkel 1991). We have already seen that there is evidence of CNS dysfunction in CFS, but whether this dysfunction causes the symptoms of the disorder or whether it is a result of behavioural changes due to the illness is still unclear. However, this is another hypothesis which is popular with CFS patients. A recent article by the editor of a support group explains:

> The areas in the brain which are most affected are
> (1) the limbic system, which functions, in part, as a processor of emotions;
> (2) the temporal lobe, in which emotion is joined to experience to facilitate memory formation.

These two areas are, of course, two of the areas in the brain most affected by CFS. Changes in neurotransmitter activity can cause depression (low serotonin levels), irritability (low followed by high serotonin levels), euphoria (high norepinephrine levels) and jitters or acute anxiety (excitatory neurotransmitters). As well as these brain generated emotional states there are of course the inevitable and natural reactions and emotional upsets and frustrations that result from not having a functioning mind or body ...

(Booth 1999a:35)

While this is a very eloquent explanation of the emotional upset in CFS, at this stage the evidence for the range of neurotransmitter dysfunction included in this description is slim.

In conclusion, depression is definitely a risk factor for the development of CFS. The most plausible explanation for this relationship at this stage is that in many patients depression interacts with other psychological and biological variables in contributing to the onset of CFS. Firm conclusions are made difficult by the fact that both CFS and depression are heterogeneous conditions and more in-depth comparisons are needed of possible underlying mechanisms in these two conditions.

Chronic fatigue syndrome and anxiety

On average around 20 per cent of CFS patients meet current criteria for an anxiety disorder (see Abbey 1996 for review). DSM III and DSM III-R diagnoses include generalised anxiety disorder (GAD), panic disorder and to a lesser extent phobic disorders. Although the point prevalence is higher than that of the general community, most studies have been unable to show a significant difference in lifetime or current anxiety disorders between CFS patients and both healthy and medical controls (Farmer et al. 1995; Johnson, DeLuca and Natelson 1996a; Katon et al. 1991).

However, a recent study using the latest DSM IV criteria found that 56.6 per cent of CFS patients met criteria for a diagnosis of GAD, compared to only 14 per cent of controls (Fischler et al. 1997a). The results from this study are probably due to the changes in the diagnostic criteria, which no longer require that GAD be excluded in the presence of a mood disorder. This suggests that previous rates of GAD in CFS may have been underestimated.

Anxiety may contribute to the experience of symptoms in CFS in a number of ways. Fatigue, myalgia and sleep disturbance are reported by the majority of patients with GAD, while headache, dizziness and chest pain characterise panic disorder. CFS patients may easily misattribute these symptoms as signs of an ongoing disease process. In addition, as discussed earlier under the organic hypotheses, hyperventilation usually associated with panic disorder may play a significant role in a subset of CFS patients. Few studies have investigated anxiety in CFS and the way in which it may contribute to symptoms warrants further attention.

Chronic fatigue syndrome and somatisation disorder

The rates for somatisation disorder are lower than those for anxiety disorder, with most studies reporting that between 10 and 20 per cent of CFS patients fulfil criteria (see Abbey 1996 for review). However, these prevalence rates are still elevated, as studies consistently show that CFS patients have significantly higher rates of somatisation when compared to other groups of medically ill patients as well as depressed patients (Fischler *et al.* 1997a; Johnson, DeLuca and Natelson 1996b; Katon *et al.* 1991).

The relevance of these findings is debatable, as the assessment of somatisation disorder in CFS poses significant problems. First, the criteria for both disorders require multiple symptoms. As such, the more symptoms that are included in the CFS definition, the more likely patients will meet criteria for somatisation. Indeed, Lane and colleagues (1991) reported that patients meeting the original CDC case definition for CFS were almost six times more likely to be diagnosed with somatisation disorder than fatigued cases who did not meet criteria. Second, criteria for somatisation disorder include the presentation of symptoms for which there is no organic explanation. If CFS symptoms are coded as physical rather than psychiatric, there is a definite drop in the number of patients meeting criteria for somatisation disorder (Johnson, DeLuca and Natelson 1996b; Lane, Manu and Matthews 1991).

Therefore, in many ways the number of CFS patients identified as having somatisation disorder can be viewed as an artefact of the specific criteria used to define both conditions. The diagnosis is probably most useful for identifying CFS patients who are most severely affected. Patients with a comorbid diagnosis of somatisation disorder report a substantially higher number of somatic symptoms, have a longer illness duration, higher rates of health care utilisation and current psychiatric morbidity (Fischler *et al.* 1997a; Hickie *et al.* 1995).

Personality and CFS

Up until now we have focused on major psychiatric or Axis I diagnoses in CFS, but abnormalities of personality or Axis II disorders have been investigated by a few CFS researchers. High rates of personality disorders, including histrionic, borderline, obsessive compulsive and avoidant have been diagnosed in CFS patients (Johnson, DeLuca and Natelson 1996c; Millon *et al.* 1989). However, they have significantly fewer Axis II diagnoses when compared to patients with major depression and cannot be distinguished from MS patients on the basis of personality disorder (Johnson, DeLuca and Natelson 1996c; Pepper *et al.*,1993). These results suggest that personality may be adversely affected by the experience of chronic illness, rather than that personality disorder leads to CFS.

Others have used self-report inventories to assess personality traits in CFS patients. Two studies using the Minnesota Multiphasic Personality Inventory (MMPI), which assesses personality traits, have reported elevated mean profiles on the hypochondriasis, depression, hysteria and neuroticism subscales (Blakely *et al.* 1991; Schmaling and Jones 1996). Substantial controversy surrounds the use of the MMPI in medically ill patients as many of the items are sensitive to physical symptoms. However, neuroticism (a tendency to be anxious, hostile, insecure and vulnerable) appears to be a stable personality trait not affected by life change (Costa *et al.* 1986). This finding suggests that certain personality traits in CFS patients may not be solely a response to the illness. It may be that these personality traits are risk factors for the development of the illness. However, a longitudinal study found that CFS patients' overall level of neuroticism was unrelated to recovery (Wilson *et al.* 1994a).

Perhaps more relevant to CFS is sufferers' personal portrayals of their premorbid personalities. CFS patients typically report that prior to their illness they were highly active, ambitious people who were constantly on the go, taking more care of others' needs than their own. It is not unusual for patients to report that they spent up to eighty hours a week working and seldom took time off for leisure or holidays. The following transcripts provide a clear illustration of this process.

> I used to do three jobs when everybody else would have been satisfied doing one. I've always driven myself quite a lot … doing loads of things … having to be all things to all people.
>
> (cited in Clements *et al.* 1997b:618)

I was an extremely energetic person. Physically I was in good shape. I was working 12–13 hours a day, including weekends, going to school nights, and teaching. I had a husband, children, kept up with the laundry, cooked on weekends for the week. Until recently, I hadn't had a vacation in years.

(cited in Ware 1993:64)

I was working probably 60 hours a week and some weeks a lot more. There wasn't enough time to get everything done. And things that needed to get done were assigned to me because my boss knew I would get them done. So he really loaded me down with a lot of stuff. And I should have said no, but I didn't, because you know, I thought, I'm superman ... In retrospect, I mean, it was really pretty dumb.

(cited in Ware 1993:64)

These premorbid accounts of personality are often used to combat claims that CFS is in any way related to psychological disorders. One sufferer writes of her GP's scepticism towards her condition:

Did he really think that someone who had been so active would just give it all up and become a neurotic individual?

(Theresa cited in Steincamp 1989:35)

In line with these self-reports, CFS patients in two retrospective analyses rated themselves as more hard driving and action prone prior to the onset of their illness than healthy controls or patients with chronic organic or psychiatric disorders (Lewis, Cooper and Bennett 1994; Van Houdenhove *et al.* 1995). A similar study found that CFS patients rated themselves as more extroverted prior to their illness (Buckley *et al.* 1999). Although these studies are subject to retrospective bias, it is possible that the tendency of many CFS patients to be achievement orientated contributes to CFS through high personal expectations. Certain negative aspects of perfectionism, such as self-doubt and parental expectations, correlate with fatigue in healthy people (Magnusson, Nias and White 1996). These characteristics of perfectionism may make people vulnerable to the stressors or triggers of CFS. Patients frequently describe how when they first get ill they do not allow themselves sufficient time to recover. At the slightest indication that their symptoms are abating they return to their premorbid rush of activity, possibly in an attempt to stave off self-doubts about their ability to perform (Surawy *et al.* 1995). As discussed in greater detail in Chapter 7, these behaviours may play an important role in perpetuating and maintaining the condition.

In summary, personality factors may contribute to CFS in a number of ways. Premorbid personality disorder may act as a risk factor for the illness in some cases. Perfectionistic traits and high personal expectations may also influence how patients initially cope with the illness. The inability to take sufficient time to recover from an acute illness episode may contribute to the chronic illness.

Chronic fatigue syndrome and stress

Although CFS patients are loath to accept psychological explanations for their illness, they often acknowledge that stress has played a role. Around 70 per cent of patients believe that stress and overwork are a significant factor in their illness (Moss-Morris 1997; Ray *et al.* 1998). However, as illustrated in the following two examples, they tend to make an important distinction: stress interacts with physical agents in causing their CFS rather than stress being a psychological cause of their illness.

> Pushing myself too hard I suppose which led me to have a very low resistance, so when the virus did come along I didn't have the resources to deal with it. So, a mixture of stress and then the organic thing coming along and me not being able to cope.
>
> (cited in Ray *et al.* 1998:104)

> Things like stress at work ... weaken the immune system ... It seems to me that perhaps a virus, not necessarily a very harmful one on its own, might get below the body's defences because of the weaknesses.
>
> (cited in Clements *et al.* 1997a:618)

Stress as a cause of chronic fatigue syndrome

The empirical evidence for the aetiological role of stress in CFS is inconsistent. One retrospective report found that CFS patients experienced significantly more life changes prior to the onset of their illness than healthy controls (Masuda *et al.* 1994), while another found no differences between CFS patients, irritable bowel syndrome patients and healthy controls on a life events checklist (Lewis and Wessely 1992).

Prospective studies have found that the experience of stressful life events is more strongly associated with the onset of psychiatric disorder and the severity of fatigue, rather than CF or CFS (Bruce-Jones *et al.* 1994; Chalder *et al.* in submission).

A limitation of these studies is their reliance on life events as a measure of stress. The term stress is more broadly applied by CFS patients to describe feelings of 'being overwhelmed by obligations and commitments, experiences of loss, fears of displeasing others, or feelings of loneliness and isolation' (Ware 1993:65). In other words, patients' personal perceptions of being overcommitted, inadequate or lonely, or both, may be more relevant than objective life events. In support of this, Lewis and colleagues (1992) found that when compared to patients with irritable bowel syndrome and healthy controls, CFS patients perceived that they had significantly poorer social support prior to their illness.

Another possible source of stress is a past history of traumatic events, which may have occurred long before the onset of CFS. Around 75 per cent of CFS patients report having been sexually or physically abused, or both, during childhood or adulthood compared to only 30 per cent of healthy controls (Schmaling and DiClementi 1995). Despite these dramatic figures, few patients seem to relate a past trauma to their CFS (Moss-Morris 1997; Ware 1993). It is also unclear at this stage if such events do indeed have an aetiological role to play. It is possible that victimisation lowers people's resistance to disease through alterations to the immune system. Alternatively, a traumatic history may make people more vulnerable to future stressors or ongoing distress, or both. This fact, coupled with a need to be seen as successful and achievement orientated, may result in the distress manifesting as somatic symptoms.

Stress as an aggravator of chronic fatigue syndrome

The experience of life events does appear to influence the course of CFS, although the effects seem to be largely mediated by the experience of emotional distress. Lutgendorf and colleagues (1995) investigated CFS patients who had recently experienced the devastating effects of a severe hurricane. Patients who had been most exposed to this disaster showed significant increases in doctor-rated relapses, self-reported symptoms and functional disability. However, patients' post-disaster distress was a much stronger predictor of these changes than the actual level of the disruption afforded by the hurricane.

Thus, patients' perceptions of stressful events rather than life events themselves may contribute to both the onset and aggravation of the condition. The experience of social adversity itself may be more strongly related to psychiatric disorder and severity of fatigue than CFS.

Summary of the psychiatric findings

In summary, prospective studies suggest that psychological factors such as premorbid distress and a past history of psychiatric illness, particularly depression, play a significant role in the development of CFS. Other factors such as anxiety, somatisation, achievement orientated personality traits, neuroticism, a past history of traumatic events and perceived stress also appear to play a role in either the onset or maintenance of the condition. While these results do not negate the likelihood that organic factors are also involved in CFS, they certainly provide convincing evidence for the role of psychological factors in this illness. Despite this, the majority of CFS patients adamantly claim that their illness is largely physical in origin. As we saw in the previous chapter, they eagerly await results from organic investigations of their illnesses, and are easily swayed by the dramatic claims of preliminary work. In contrast, they ridicule any psychological findings from even well-designed research studies. In the following sections we explore some of the reasons behind these illness beliefs.

The social stigma of psychiatric disorder

Society's attitude towards people with psychiatric disorder may be one of the key reasons for patients' reluctance to accept psychological explanations for their illness. As we saw in Chapter 1, the very existence of fatigue syndromes has rested on their recognition as organic conditions. Once these syndromes are viewed as primarily psychiatric in nature they tend to fall from favour and are seldom diagnosed by the medical profession. Thus, in many ways Western society's attitude towards psychiatry reflects the 'either–or' thinking of the medical profession: if symptoms are not viewed as entirely physical they must be psychological, which also implies that they are less acceptable. Once a somatic illness is seen to be psychological, the assumption is frequently made by patients and doctors alike that the symptoms are imaginary (Ware 1993; Wessely 1990). These beliefs are cogently portrayed in the following excerpt from an article written by a CFS sufferer:

Misdiagnosing ME as all in the mind is extremely damaging. It precludes helping patients find appropriate physical treatment; leads to perilous advice to snap out of it and exercise; kills doctor–patient trust dead; stops research before it has started; and leaves the patient feeling alone and misunderstood, self-doubting and doubted by others ... Whereas a physical disease is external and happens to us, leaving the 'us' intact, a psychological label at the best of times can be seen as imputing personal weakness or blame, putting in question the whole viability of the self.

(Thompson 1992:26)

Another patient told us that she no longer consulted conventional medical practitioners as they refused to acknowledge the reality of her condition:

I think people with physical CFS need more doctors' support and people to believe in them instead of thinking it's in the head. People need plenty of support, they didn't want to have CFS. I have found that some doctors can utterly destroy your self confidence and I never want to see another one again.

For patients, therefore, a psychological diagnosis not only invalidates the extent of their suffering, but it is seen as a direct insult to their sense of self. This attitude that a physical disease is more 'valid and deserving' than a psychological one pervades the current media coverage of CFS, and the illness is almost always presented to the public as being caused by a specific pathological agent (MacLean and Wessely 1994). The opinion that people with depression are just unmotivated, lazy individuals is not uncommon and the lay CFS literature is full of such inaccurate stereotypes. The president of a prominent ME association writes of CFS patients, 'they almost have too much will power, whereas depressives have virtually none' (Dowsett 1990). Similarly, a recent ME fact sheet contained the following explanation of 'why ME is not just depression':

Endogenously depressed patients are lonely, hopeless and helpless, while the ME patient will only admit to being discouraged. The depressed patient has no future and is anhedonistic; but the patient with ME will beg for treatment because this disease is slowing them down, interfering with plans and life. While depressives are phlegmatic and withdrawn, the ME attitude is positive and hopeful.

With these attitudes it is not surprising that a psychiatric label is something to be avoided. Not only do physical attributions protect people from self-blame, but they also avoid society's disdain.

Patients' experiences of medical attitudes

These 'either–or' attitudes towards illness are also prevalent in the medical profession. One doctor is even quoted as saying 'ME is an imaginary disease ... for which the best treatment is psychiatric' (Herbert 1986, cited in Steincamp 1989:5). Certainly, a number of CFS patients report that doctors do not believe their symptoms are real and that they encounter either considerable scorn or a patronising attitude in medical consultations (Broom and Woodward 1996; Cooper 1997).

> He told me I had a bizarre range of symptoms, that he'd never heard of anything like that. It had to be in my head – was I finding it difficult to cope with the beginning of the school holidays ... I thought if I was going crazy and I didn't feel like I was going crazy, then I must have been really crazy! I had to be very mentally disturbed to have made my body that sick!
>
> (cited in Broom and Woodward 1996: 370)

> At the time I was so depressed because nobody was helping me ... I found it awfully upsetting in the health service, you know a lot of arrogance and misunderstanding of what I was saying to them. I felt at some point that I was sort of treated as if it was my fault.
>
> (cited in Ax et al. 1997:252)

Women patients in particular report that their physical symptoms are disregarded by doctors in favour of their emotional distress (Broom and Woodward 1996; Cooper 1997). One young woman explains how her doctor was only interested in her emotional state:

> When I saw her I was feeling so tired, depressed, unworthy, self doubting, confused, that I am sure I simply convinced her that the problem was emotional. However, these feelings were entirely suited to someone with an undiagnosed, becoming chronic, physical–mental organic illness. I argued with her asserting the validity of my physical symptoms, only to be told that these were being used by me as a prop to opt out of life! I soon stopped arguing ... She wasn't

offensive in her manner – very gentle actually. She obviously thought she knew what was best for me, regardless of my input. This was probably the most degrading aspect of the exchange, which I found devastating on top of everything else …

(cited in Broom and Woodward 1996:370)

Other CFS sufferers describe negative experiences with psychiatric health professionals and it is not uncommon for the self-help literature to include advice on how to survive a psychiatric encounter. One CFS sufferer describes her encounters with a range of health professionals:

I stopped pushing myself. It had become more and more apparent that the more I pushed myself the worse I got. But I couldn't get any medical back up for this point of view. And I've seen several doctors and psychiatric workers and … one psychiatric worker who was just disgusting, absolutely disgusting. So I think it's actually put me off the psychiatric point of view.

(cited in Ax *et al.* 1997:252)

Some patients do report positive encounters with health professionals. Invariably, these health professionals acknowledged the patient's suffering and the reality of their illness:

He is a wonderful doctor, a lovely, lovely man and without him I don't think I would have been able to take it, I really don't … on the very first day I saw him I said 'Do you think I am ill?' And he said 'yes', and I tapped my head and said 'Do you think it is all in here?' And he said 'No – I can see you are ill!' And, of course, then he knew I was ill and he went out of his way to treat me.

(cited in Broom and Woodward 1996:201)

However, in general, CFS patients' experiences of medical encounters suggest that health professionals often do not take their illness seriously. Many doctors seem to have difficulties with illnesses that do not fit neatly under the psychiatric or biological umbrellas. A patient who presents to a doctor with a self-diagnosis of CFS is likely to be regarded as someone who takes up too much time and poses a difficult management problem (Scott *et al.* 1998). With such negation of their illness experience it is not hard to understand why CFS patients so desperately seek the single organic test which will prove the existence of their symptoms.

The adamant rejection of psychological causation can be seen as an attempt to obtain medical and social validation for their suffering.

Medical attitudes towards diagnosis and treatment of CFS

Doctors' attitudes towards CFS are also reflected in their reluctance to diagnose the condition. It is not uncommon for CFS patients to be ill for quite some time before they receive a medical label for their complaints:

> It was three years before we knew it was ME. As first we clutched onto everything that might be a diagnosis and no doctor could tell us what was wrong.
>
> (cited in Cooper 1997:195)

Not having a label on which to hang their symptoms is often a confusing and distressing experience for patients:

> I would come out very confused. I went to see him because I knew I should take time off work as I was so sick. But he kept saying you are looking well and he would praise the way I had been living my life, the way I was striving to be fit and keep working … It really did me in the long run.
>
> (cited in Broom and Woodward 1996:373)

Most patients describe the process of receiving a diagnosis as a relief (Ax *et al.* 1997). One study reported that 86 per cent of CFS patients felt they were sicker during the time they were ill but had no label for their illness (Broom and Woodward 1996). A label often provides patients with something concrete to tackle:

> I felt better for the diagnosis because for the first time I really felt in myself 'now I can do something about this'. I knew what I was up against and what I could do.
>
> Diagnosis was a release because up until then I kept struggling to work and struggling to keep going. It changed the way I lived my life then. And when I stopped pushing so hard I started to get a bit better. I stopped worrying what society thought.
>
> (cited in Broom and Woodward 1996:373)

A diagnosis also legitimates the suffering.

> It [diagnosis] made it a lot better. I'd actually got something I could hang onto. At least I had something to definitely say this person is really ill. I already knew I had a chronic illness … it was just a matter of somebody accepting that I really had a problem.
>
> (cited in Ax *et al.* 1997:252)

Why then are doctors so reluctant to diagnose CFS? For many doctors a diagnosis of CFS is seen to have negative rather than positive consequences for the patient. They worry that the lack of explanation and specific treatment for CFS will result in patients remaining sick once they have been diagnosed (Broom and Woodward 1996). However, this does not appear to be in the patients' best interest and possibly reflects doctors' feelings of helplessness if they cannot provide a definite biological treatment. Indeed, it is not uncommon for doctors to give CFS patients the message that there is nothing they can do for them. One CFS patient went back to her doctor for advice after receiving a diagnosis of CFS:

> I went back to the doctor and she said she couldn't help. I asked 'where do I go from here?' and she just shrugged her shoulders and said there was nothing she could do really.
>
> (cited in Cooper 1997:199)

Nevertheless, there are things doctors can do to help CFS patients cope better with their illness and improve their quality of life. While this approach is different from the traditional curative stance taken by many doctors, as we will discuss in detail in the final chapter, these management strategies can make a substantial difference. Central to this approach is the adoption of a multifactorial cognitive behavioural model of the illness.

Cognitive behavioural models of chronic fatigue syndrome

Wessely and colleagues (1991) proposed the formative cognitive behavioural model of CFS. They suggested that an organic insult such as a virus precipitates a cycle of psychological responses, which mediate between the acute organic illness and the chronic syndrome. In other words, while organic factors might precipitate the illness, cognitive behavioural factors perpetuate the condition. Wessely and colleagues explain that when resuming normal activity levels following a bad viral infection, it is common to experience symptoms of physical deconditioning. If people attribute these symptoms to signs of ongoing disease rather than deconditioning, they will tend to resort to rest and inactivity in an attempt to 'cure' the symptoms. A cycle of avoidance and symptom experience develops which can lead to loss of control, demoralisation and possibly depression and anxiety. These psychological states can further perpetuate the illness through generating more physical symptoms and possibly through compromising the immune system.

Surawy *et al.* (1995) expanded this earlier formulation to include an explanation of predisposing factors. They suggest that predisposed people are highly achievement orientated and base their self-esteem and respect from others on their ability to live up to certain high standards. When such people are faced with precipitating factors which affect their ability to perform, such as a combination of excessive stress and an acute illness, their initial reaction is to press on and keep coping. This behaviour leads to exhaustion. In making sense of the situation a physical attribution for the exhaustion is made, which protects their self-esteem by avoiding the suggestion that their inability to cope is a sign of personal weakness. Physical attributions result in people focusing on the somatic rather than emotional aspects of their illness. Symptoms which could be physiological concomitants of chronic psychological distress or inactivity, or both, such as fatigue, poor concentration and muscle pain are interpreted as signs of an ongoing disease. This somatic interpretive bias leads to a perpetuating cycle of avoidance of activity in an attempt to reduce symptoms. However, reduced activity conflicts with achievement orientation and may result in bursts of activity in an attempt to meet expectations. These periodic bursts of activity inevitably exacerbate symptoms and result in failure, which further reinforces the belief that they have a serious illness. As time goes by efforts to meet previous standards of achievement are abandoned and patients become increasingly preoccupied with their symptoms and illness. This results in chronic disability and the belief that one has an ongoing incurable illness.

These models incorporate a range of factors which have been shown to be important in CFS illness. They take into account how predisposing psychiatric illness or personality factors, or both, have a role to play as well as stress and biological factors such as viruses. These cognitive behavioural models, though they provide a useful guide for interventions, can be criticised for not elaborating on the way in which some of the psychological factors may interact with the biological concomitants of CFS such as alterations to the HPA. In the following three chapters we provide more detailed psychological models of the factors which help to perpetuate CFS. We also provide a review of the empirical support for these models and in the final chapter we discuss how this information can be used to improve the quality of life of CFS sufferers. It is important to note, before reading these chapters, that the models presented here are drawn from health psychology. They are not exclusive to CFS and have been developed to explain the way in which patients or people in general interpret symptom information and adapt to their illnesses. In other words, these models do not preclude a biological basis to CFS, rather they provide a psychological explanation of some of the factors involved in the chronicity of the condition.

Chapter 5

Making sense of symptoms in chronic fatigue syndrome

At any one time there are a great many people with physical symptoms. These range from minor coughs and colds to more severe and threatening symptoms. How people interpret physical symptoms and seek help for them is a fascinating aspect of human behaviour. Common sense would suggest that people who seek help for their symptoms are suffering from more severe symptoms than those who do not seek medical attention. However, research shows that this is incorrect. People's interpretation of symptoms and their help-seeking behaviour is determined by a large number of factors aside from physiological activity and symptom severity.

Symptoms and bodily sensations are often difficult to interpret. A person experiencing chest pain might ask themselves, 'Is this indigestion or is it the first sign of a heart attack?' People have a limited ability to work out what is going on in their body and so they tend to rely on other factors to make judgements about symptoms. Here illness beliefs, past experience and external information can be helpful in deciding whether a symptom is transitory or serious. In the case of chest pain, a person who regularly experiences heartburn and who has just eaten a large meal may be more likely to see the symptom as transitory than a person who does not have these immediate and past experiences.

Symptom perception has a great deal of relevance to CFS as these patients report suffering from a large number and wide variety of symptoms. In one study we conducted, CFS patients reported the type of symptoms they experience 'all the time' or 'frequently' (Moss-Morris 1997). Not surprisingly the most frequently endorsed symptom is fatigue after any exercise, followed by poor concentration and forgetfulness. However, other symptoms are also very common. As can be seen in Figure 5.1, a large number of CFS patients report muscle pain and stiff or

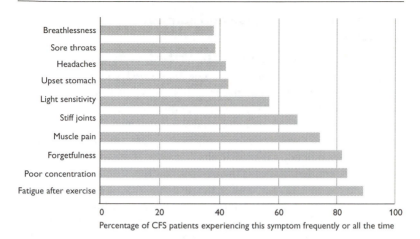

Figure 5.1 Reported symptoms of CFS patients.

sore joints. Rates of other symptoms are also high in this group with sore throat, nausea and headaches being particularly frequent.

In fact, CFS patients report a wider range of symptoms than do patients with rheumatoid arthritis, cardiac disease or depression (Moss-Morris 1997; Weinman *et al.* 1996). It is not only the number but also the extent of the symptoms and fatigue which patients find so debilitating. One of our CFS participants described the nature of CFS-related fatigue:

> This is not just a tiredness but a profound weakness which words cannot describe, and it is so incapacitating one can virtually do nothing to fight back. One can only lie and wait until the extreme weakness has lifted. Both mental and physical energy is at an all time low.

Another patient described the devastating effect of activity on the experience of symptoms:

> When I push myself physically I 'crash'. I lose all strength, my muscles and joints become extremely painful which no drug can ease. I feel dizzy and shaky and my sinuses become extremely sore. I lose my appetite and feel nauseous. The only way I can help this is to go to bed. I usually spend a week in bed. After that I find any physical activity makes me feel weak and exhausted e.g. changing chairs, having a shower. I go to bed early and sleep in the afternoon. I can hardly concentrate at all.

The prevalence of fatigue and somatic symptoms in the community

Although the accounts of fatigue in CFS are very dramatic, fatigue symptoms are not restricted to people diagnosed with CFS. In fact, fatigue is one of the most commonly reported symptoms. Typically, 20 to 40 per cent of participants in general population studies report feeling tired or fatigued all the time (Lewis and Wessely 1992). In primary practice samples, the rates are even higher. A recent study, conducted in 1,000 primary practice patients, found 67 per cent of women and 45 per cent of men reported fatigue in the past month (Kroenke 1998). For 5–10 per cent of patients, fatigue will be the principal reason for the consultation (Cathebras *et al.* 1992). A large community study found that only a small minority of people reporting excessive fatigue met criteria for CFS (Pawlikowska *et al.* 1994). However, they did not find a qualitative difference in the fatigue experienced and concluded that CFS exists at the end of a continuum of fatigue severity rather than being a distinct entity.

Other CFS symptoms are also common in the community, with 36 per cent of primary care patients reporting headache, 34 per cent insomnia, and 59 per cent joint or limb pain (Kroenke 1998). General population surveys also show that during any two-week period up to 30 per cent of people complain of muscle aches and pains, 38 per cent of headache, and 16 per cent of sleep disturbance (Dunnell and Cartwright 1972; Hannay 1978). While it may be logical to assume that these symptom reports are a result of biological processes, there is now substantial evidence to show that how individuals interpret bodily sensations and symptoms is strongly affected by psychological processes.

Interpreting symptoms

At any one time, we are processing an enormous amount of somatic information but we only have a small attentional capacity. While you are sitting reading this, you are processing information from your legs and back. Unless your attention is drawn to these sensations or you have some reason to be monitoring them, then these sensations are processed automatically and unconsciously. Various processes can alter the way we monitor such sensations. One important factor is how much is happening in the surrounding environment.

Situational factors

When attention is focussed externally, less focus is maintained on internal sensations, so individuals placed in boring situations tend to report more symptoms than those in stimulating or interesting environments. People who live alone, are socially isolated, and who work in the house, as opposed to those in paid employment, tend to report more symptoms (Pennebaker 1982). Most of us have had the experience of being engrossed in a sporting or other activity and being unaware until later of a cut or injury that has occurred.

Any situational factor that raises the awareness of symptoms or illness promotes their recognition by individuals. So when a friend you have just had lunch with suddenly feels ill, this is likely to set up a search for similar symptoms consistent with your friend's illness. Studies have shown that individuals are very susceptible to noticing symptoms in this way. There are a number of real life examples of this. A common one in the environment we work in is 'medical students' disease'. Here, students studying the symptoms of an illness focus on their own internal states, and symptoms consistent with the illness they are studying tend to emerge. In a medical school class, typically about a third of students will by their third year admit to this phenomenon, with a number commonly self-diagnosing (incorrectly) a brain tumour, heart attack or multiple sclerosis.

On a community-wide level, this process can be seen in a dramatic form in mass psychogenic illness. This is the shared occurrence of a group of similar symptoms in a cohesive social setting for which there is no plausible pathological explanation. In most cases individuals present with ambiguous symptoms, typically headache, cough, pain, rash, dizziness and nausea that develop in response to a threatening experience such as a strong odour or perceived toxin. There are some dramatic examples of mass psychogenic illness such as an epidemic that occurred in a group of over 1,000 naval recruits housed in common barracks (Struewing and Gray 1990). All developed at least one new symptom over a ten-hour period, and 375 were evacuated to hospital. There was a perception of an airborne toxin among recruits and medical personnel. Air sample testing and laboratory findings were unremarkable. Most recruits transported from the scene improved quickly without specific therapy. Similar dramatic episodes of fatigue-like illnesses, such as the Royal Free epidemic, were also described in Chapter 1.

Mental schemas

The influence of mental schemas on symptom reports usually works more subtly, such as in studies where individuals have been given a false disease diagnosis. This has occurred in two different types of study. In some studies, participants in health screening programmes such as blood pressure screening have been incorrectly labelled as having hypertension. When these subjects were followed up they were found to have higher levels of absenteeism and poorer self-appraisals of their health and lower subjective well-being than non-labelled individuals (Bloom and Monterossa 1981; Haynes *et al.* 1978).

Other studies have investigated this phenomenon more directly. One group of researchers has given false information to subjects after a saliva test and told some subjects that they had an enzyme deficiency that makes them susceptible to a pancreatic disorder (Croyle and Sande 1988; Jemmott, Ditto and Croyle 1986). In these studies, participants falsely labelled with the deficiency tend to report more symptoms than those not labelled. When asked, labelled participants also recalled more behaviours that supposedly increased the risk of the deficiency syndrome.

These findings are consistent with Leventhal's symmetry rule (Leventhal, Meyer and Nerenz 1980) which proposes that when given a diagnostic label, an individual will seek symptoms consistent with the diagnosis. This rule also works the other way around, so when an individual has symptoms, he or she will seek a diagnostic label to explain the condition. An example of how this could work in CFS is when someone may experience extreme fatigue over a period of time and is motivated to look for a diagnostic label. Once the individual has been given the diagnostic label of CFS, he or she is more likely to notice symptoms consistent with this label. Because many CFS patients associate a wide range of symptoms with the illness, it is easy to understand how they could assume that any sensation they experience is a sign of their illness.

One sufferer explains some of the bizarre bodily sensations and symptoms she associates with CFS:

> ... shooting pain developing into persistent aching ... irritability caused by noise or light, blurring of vision, memory loss and trouble with forming the mental images and words ... loss of sensation (so one is less aware of injury), pins and needles, taste loss/strange tastes (especially metallic ones), taste/smell magnified, visual annoyance

caused by dots or stripes, vertigo, sudden balance loss ... cold in warm weather, and perspire in the cold ...

(Horne 1992:17)

Others may interpret signs and symptoms of normal processes such as ageing or lack of sleep to their illness. For instance, one patient told us:

Ever since I have had ME I wake up with black rings around my eyes. I only wore glasses for driving because I am short sighted. Now the world's a blur and I wear them all the time.

Therefore, once one has the label of CFS, symptoms are likely to be interpreted as signs of an ongoing disease process. This in itself generates concern and an increased vigilance for new symptoms.

The schematic processing of illness information may also interact with situational factors in increasing the experience of symptoms. Patients with CFS tend to reduce their levels of activity in response to their fears that the symptoms they are experiencing signal that their illness is getting worse. This has the potential to decrease the amount of external stimulation CFS patients are exposed to, which will result in them becoming more internally focussed.

The influence of distress on symptoms

An important factor that is closely related to the reporting of physical symptoms is psychological distress. Psychological distress incorporates the concepts of depression, anxiety or negative affect. We have already seen in Chapter 4 that premorbid distress is a predicator of CFS and that CFS patients have higher levels of distress than a number of other chronic illness groups. Distress in CFS is strongly associated with the experience of somatic symptoms (Wessely et al. 1996a). This relationship is true both for symptoms included in the current CDC definition of CFS and non-CDC somatic symptoms. Therefore the association between distress and symptoms has particular relevance for CFS.

Individuals who score high on measures of psychological distress tend to report more physical symptom complaints in all situations. There is considerable research now showing psychological distress is related to symptom reporting but not to organic disease (Costa et al. 1986; Watson and Pennebaker 1989). Much of the evidence suggests that reports of symptoms and distress are closely interrelated. Some researchers in this area have gone so far as to question whether symptom reports are actually a better measure of emotional distress than health.

This is not to say the symptoms are 'hypochondriacal' or 'all in the head', but psychological distress can cause more physiological activity because individuals are worked-up, upset or worried. Distress can also change the way we look at things so we make more negative interpretations of symptoms that may arise. We have shown that both CFS and depressed patients tend to interpret the meaning of symptoms in a more negative way than do healthy controls (Moss-Morris and Petrie 1997).

Anxiety can also make us more alert to other physical problems. If a new symptom is detected, it is more likely to be interpreted as a sign of an illness than if it was thought to be a normal response to a stressful situation (Moss-Morris and Petrie 1999). Distress and bad moods also influence self-reports of health and symptoms. From studies where mood has been manipulated in a laboratory situation, we know that people in a positive mood rate themselves as healthier and report fewer symptoms. However, people in negative moods report more symptoms, are more pessimistic that any actions they take would relieve their symptoms, and perceive themselves as more vulnerable to future illness (Salovey *et al.* 1991). Similar findings are made if people undergo induction techniques to make them more self-focussed. Increased self-focus leads to an increase in symptom reports, suggesting that negative mood may operate through the process of heightened awareness of the self (Ingram 1990).

In most cases CFS patients have a very different explanation for the relationship between distress and symptoms. They tend to view their psychological distress as a symptom in itself and an indication of the ongoing disease process. One patient explains:

> Mood swings and tendencies to overreactions occur. Hidden parts of the personality show and negative feelings arise as the illness progresses.
>
> (Horne 1992:17)

Thus, for patients, the experience of distress reinforces their schema of having an ongoing, uncontrollable illness.

Distress can also influence the way in which people perceive the state of their bodies in general. This can be illustrated with respect to the immune system. Over the past few years the immune system has gathered increased prominence in public discourse about health and illness. It is seen by the public as the key to avoiding many illnesses including cancer. The immune system is also popularly seen as being weakened by the stresses of modern life and many CFS patients see an ineffective immune system as the cause of their symptoms. One of our CFS participants told us:

> My immune system is definitely affected to a large degree, causing continual sinus and throat problems and also sore glands. Also I have not had a cold for eight years. The logic of this seems to escape most doctors.

Many remedies are promoted to CFS patients and the public in general as ways of boosting the immune system. One women with CFS describes her attempts to improve her health:

> I take spirulina by the handful and balase blue green algae. I also take *Ginkgo biloba* and garlic to boost my immune system.

A visit to any health food shop or even supermarket provides an opportunity to see the vast number and variety of products claiming to enhance immunity. It is an interesting psychological problem to consider how people come to believe their immune system needs upgrading when we do not have direct information on how our immune system is functioning.

In a recent study, we found individuals are not at all accurate in perceiving the state of their immune system. Perceptions of immune function were actually unrelated to various immune markers but closely related to mood and in particular, feelings of fatigue and vigour. The experience of recent physical symptoms, while not as strong as mood variables, were also important in perceptions of immune functioning (Petrie *et al.* 1999). So individuals who are feeling fatigued and who have had recent symptoms are likely to blame their immune system for their condition.

Laboratory studies of symptoms in CFS

The concepts discussed so far in this chapter can be used to explain the findings from laboratory studies which have attempted to provide objective evidence of neuropsychological and fatigue symptoms in CFS. The neuropsychological studies have used standard measures to quantify the extent of the memory and attention deficit in CFS patients. Taken together the results of these studies suggest that CFS patients are slower to process information than healthy controls and that this is reflected in their performance on more complex tasks of memory and concentration (Moss-Morris *et al.* 1996a; Wearden and Appleby 1996). However, the most consistent finding is that this deficit is out of proportion with patients' self-reports of neuropsychological difficulties. Around 75 per cent of CFS patients report concentration and memory difficulties, while only 25 per cent are rated as impaired by neuropsychological experts (Grafman *et al.* 1993; McDonald, Cope and David 1993a). Studies which have measured subjective performance have invariably found no relationship between objective test results and subjective complaints (Altay *et al.* 1990; Cope *et al.* 1995; Ray, Phillips and Weir 1993a). Rather, as with the general literature on distress and symptom reports, subjective reports of impairment in CFS have been consistently related to higher levels of psychopathology, anxiety, depression and somatic complaints (Cope *et al.* 1995; Grafman *et al.* 1993; McDonald *et al.* 1993a).

Similarly, the complaint of increased mental and physical fatigue during testing has not been substantiated. The time an individual spends on a particular test does not appear to influence CFS patients more than controls (McDonald *et al.* 1993a; Scheffers *et al.* 1992), with patients able to tolerate up to three hours of testing (Joyce, Blumenthal and Wessely 1996). Despite the fact that CFS patients often complain that the effects of fatigue are delayed until the day afterwards, a study which tested patients over a two-day period found no effects of fatigue on performance (Marshal *et al.* 1997). In fact, patients' performance showed a significant improvement on the second day of testing. Similar findings have been obtained from exercise studies which have consistently demonstrated normal muscular strength but an increased perception of effort in CFS patients (Lawrie *et al.* 1997).

These studies suggest that CFS sufferers' experience of both mental and muscle fatigue are more convincingly related to disturbances in subjective perceptions than actual abnormalities. While it could be argued that these discrepancies in perception occur because laboratory data is not a true measure of people's day-to-day experiences, similar findings have been reported in a naturalistic setting. A study using an ambulatory monitor to record the activity levels of children with CFS and matched healthy controls in their home environment, found no differences in the activity levels of these two groups (Fry and Martin 1996a). However, in this study CFS patients reported substantial fatigue and greatly reduced activity levels.

What is the explanation for CFS sufferers underestimating their activity levels and overestimating their symptoms? One suggestion is that patients with CFS have a dysfunction affecting perceptual threshold (Lloyd, Hickie and Gandevia 1988a). In other words, CFS sufferers have a reduced threshold for perceiving effort, fatigue and pain. While this explanation could account for exercise studies which have found that patients have an over-exaggerated perception of their exertion, it cannot fully explain the discrepancies in the neuropsychological studies as there is no sensory component to the perception of cognitive difficulty (Fry and Martin 1996b). An abnormal perception of effort is also unable to account for the fact that children with CFS underestimate their activity levels, nor can it explain the fact that the children's parents made similar judgement errors (Fry and Martin 1996a).

Another possibility is that CFS sufferers may report elevated levels of fatigue because their actual sensation of what is normal is out of proportion with what they believe they have achieved. CFS patients frequently describe themselves as having high expectations of themselves and as being hard-driving perfectionists. While a distorted perception of what is actually achieved can explain the disturbance in subjective reports, it does not fully account for the fact that neuropsychological studies have documented objective impairment in attentional processes.

A further contributing factor may be that CFS sufferers have a bias to monitor somatic-related information. As we have seen, heightened attention to the body increases symptom reports even in healthy people. It may be that patients with CFS have a propensity to focus on bodily sensations, which contributes to both their high symptom reports and a tendency to misinterpret bodily sensations as signs of illness or harm. Such an attention bias would help to explain the objective difficulties found when they are asked to complete tasks that require greater levels of attention. If an increased amount of CFS patients' attention is inadvertently focussed on their bodily symptoms, it is reasonable to assume that less attention will be available for other tasks. Impaired attentional processes will in turn affect the speed of processing and working memory functions. The dramatic way in which this cognitive difficulty is then interpreted may be particularly pathogenic. For instance, one CFS sufferer reports:

> This intellectual impairment is truly bizarre; we have trouble making memories, our IQ scores fall ... we have trouble finding words or our way home, we forget names of our friends and even our children.
>
> (Iverson cited in Freese 1991:ii)

This vivid description is out of proportion to the only minor difficulties found on tasks requiring high levels of attention. It is also inconsistent with the frequent finding of no impairment to higher cognitive functions or global intellectual abilities in CFS patients (Moss-Morris *et al.* 1996a; Wearden and Appleby 1996). Thus, a combination of distress, high personal expectations, inaccurate perceptions of normal performance and somatic focus may result in the dramatisation of the meaning of minor impairments.

Catastrophising about symptoms

Support for this dramatic or catastrophic style of interpreting symptoms in CFS has been obtained in two of our studies (Moss-Morris and Petrie 1997; Petrie *et al.* 1995). Catastrophising is an expectation of a highly exaggerated negative outcome far beyond what may normally be anticipated. Such a cognitive style is important in CFS because of its relationship to activity. CFS sufferers who believe that increased activity will cause a severe relapse or total body failure are more likely to stay in bed and be careful to conserve their energy.

We investigated the role of catastrophising in CFS in a large study of 282 CFS sufferers. In an open-ended question we asked patients what they thought would be the consequence of pushing themselves beyond their present physical state (Petrie *et al.* 1995). While almost all patients believed that exertion would have negative consequences for their symptoms, one-third had highly exaggerated or catastrophic expectations. Examples of catastrophic responses to the question were as follows:

> Disastrous! Putting me in a semi-paralysed state, bedridden for weeks or months at a time. Been there done that!

> Complete collapse and possibly relapse to total bedridden condition as experienced in early days of the illness.

> I would very quickly find myself in a relapse of my ME and would have to go to bed to recover and I would be totally incapacitated by it, not even having enough energy to move, speak or eat.

> I would have a stroke and die.

The results showed that while catastrophisers were not significantly different in terms of their age or number of health centre visits for CFS, they

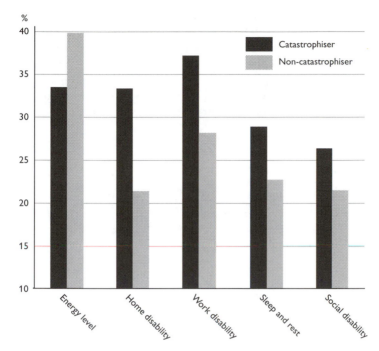

Figure 5.2 Disability in catastrophiser and non-catastrophiser CFS groups.

did differ markedly in terms of their level of disability. CFS sufferers who catastrophised about the results of pushing themselves beyond their present state had lower energy levels and were significantly more disabled in a range of activities. The results of this study, illustrated in Figure 5.2, show CFS sufferers to have higher levels of disability across a range of activities including social relations and ability to work.

This research raises the question: are catastrophisers accurate in their expectations from increased activity and does the evidence show that CFS patients have significant worsening of symptoms following activity? Not according to studies that have exposed CFS patients to mentally and physically strenuous activities over two-day periods. These studies showed increased activity actually to have a positive effect on both mood and symptoms as well as improvements on cognitive testing (Lloyd *et al.* 1994; Marshal *et al.* 1997).

The research data then shows catastrophising about symptoms to be a particularly dysfunctional coping strategy for CFS sufferers. Similar findings have been reported for chronic pain and rheumatoid arthritis patients (Keefe *et al.* 1989; Smith *et al.* 1986; Smith *et al.* 1988). Not only does catastrophising seem to lead to greater levels of distress but it also seems to severely limit daily activities. It is therefore reasonable to expect catastrophic expectations following physical exertion to be associated with a more adverse illness trajectory. Catastrophising also provides a potent example of how patients' expectations and beliefs can directly influence outcome in CFS.

Modernity and symptoms

A great deal of attention in the media and current discourse concerns the threats posed by modern life and a current fascination with health. This is seen in the number of books and television programmes now devoted to health issues. Looking around in any magazine or book store it is hard not to notice how many magazines and new book titles are devoted entirely to health issues. Other popular magazine titles frequently run health features or health scares as lead articles. Health titles also frequently appear in the bestseller lists.

From time to time, specific health scares also hit the headlines. Such stories as the risks from saccharine, fluoridation, benzene in Perrier, or the dangers of amalgam fillings appear for some days in the media and then disappear to be replaced by a new health concern. The overall effect of such stories is to undermine people's perceptions of their own health. In fact, newspaper and other stories are now much more focussed on threats to health than they have been at any time in our history.

This increase in health stories in the media has a number of effects. One important outcome is that people see themselves as vulnerable from many features of modern life. Current diets are seen as having too many additives or genetically modified substances. The air and water we drink is seen as containing pollutants that may cause illness. Threats are also perceived in new features of modern life such as electromagnetic emissions from mobile phones, power lines, computers, microwaves and radio towers.

These community concerns have been reflected in illnesses with new labels such as 'multiple chemical sensitivity', 'immune system dysfunction', 'electric allergy', 'total allergy syndrome', and 'twentieth-century disease'. All of these illnesses have in common the attribution that illness was caused by an external factor brought on by the stresses or features of modern life. Due to the increase in attention given to threats to health, people's subjective feelings of health have declined over this century. Ironically, at the same time, objective indices of health such as life expectancy have improved.

Concerns about the environment can strongly influence people's perceptions about symptoms. For example, residents with environmental concerns report two to three times more symptoms in response to an environmental scare than residents without such concerns (Roht *et al.* 1985). These situations demonstrate that, when activated by the situation, our beliefs guide the monitoring of somatic information to look for confirmatory evidence.

Another study that illustrates this process is a study of symptom prevalence and worry about high voltage transmission lines (McMahan and Meyer 1995). This study looked at people living adjacent to overhead transmission lines or one block away. There was no difference in symptoms between these two groups; however, those respondents most worried about the presence of transmission lines were more likely to report symptoms. In this study, the level of worry, rather than proximity, was most associated with symptoms. It is also the case that publicity through the media of environmental concerns in a community may set up a mental schema of what symptoms to look for and cause individuals to use this schema to evaluate their own symptoms. This can result in an over-reporting of symptoms in groups who may have no exposure (Fone, Constantine and McCloskey 1998) and an overestimation recall bias when people are asked to recall symptoms of environmental exposure (Hopwood and Guidotti 1988).

Another effect of the way modern media deals with health stories is highlighting unusual events and downplaying common causes of illness. Articles in the media concerning environmental issues often misrepresent the scientific evidence and increase public concern (Frost, Frank and Maibach 1997; Jauchem 1992). For example, there is a perception that much of the cancer today is caused by environmental pollution or artificial additives in foods. Individuals' perceptions of the causes of cancer have been influenced strongly by stories in the media which highlight artificial and environmental substances that cause cancer but neglect diet and lifestyle factors that are more commonly associated with the disease.

Modernity and CFS symptoms

Environmental concerns often form a large part of CFS patients' worries about symptoms. Many CFS sufferers blame environmental toxins either for the disease or for its exacerbation. As a corollary of this belief, some treatments for CFS have relied on reversing the effect of environmental contamination. One CFS patient comments:

> Mercury toxicity from dental amalgams made a significant contribution to my illness. Three years ago I had all my fillings replaced in conjunction with chelation therapy. Fluorescent lights, coal smoke, petrol fumes, perfume and cigarette smoke make my illness worse.

Another CFS patient states:

> There is no doubt that pollution plays a large part in making me worse. I have suffered from chemical poisoning very severely. I do not know whether my immune system has been affected by pesticide before I contracted the CFS virus or after due to a weakened immune system. I am still badly knocked about by chemicals and am having treatment to clear the CFS symptoms and toxins.

Patients also make daily decisions about symptoms based on their expectations of environmental hazards. A patient recently told us that her gums had receded 4mm overnight after city council workers had been spraying weeds outside her home.

Environmental concerns and worries can interact with psychological distress to make the development of CFS and allergies more common. Studies have demonstrated that individuals who have a history of anxiety or depression are more likely to develop medically unexplained allergy to common environmental agents (Simon, Katon and Sparks 1990) and also CFS after common viral illnesses (Wessely *et al.* 1995). These provide an example of how both physical and psychological factors, given the right circumstances, can conspire to establish functionally debilitating conditions.

As we have seen in this chapter, the process of making sense of symptoms is complex and is influenced by a range of factors outside physiological activity. While this does not negate a role for biological factors, situational and emotional factors clearly play a central role in this process. CFS is an example of a modern illness where a number of concerns about environment and strong illness perceptions have a considerable impact on the number and type of symptoms reported. In the next chapter we look at how illness beliefs are organised and how these form a critical role in the CFS syndrome.

Chapter 6

Illness representations and chronic fatigue syndrome

Imagine having an illness that was caused by a mystery virus. Your illness has a large number of severe and fluctuating symptoms that stop you from working or keeping up your normal activities. There is no cure for your condition and you are destined to live with this illness for the rest of your life. The effect of the illness on your life is likely to be profound. Not only will it affect your financial and work life, it will also make a satisfying social and intimate life difficult.

By imagining this illness you are 'trying on' many of the perceptions of illness held by CFS sufferers. We know from many areas of psychology that cognitive factors, or the way people think about things, can have a profound effect on their emotions and coping strategies. The same holds for the way individuals think about illness. In this chapter we examine how perceptions of CFS can have a strong influence on how well individuals cope with the disorder. We review the theoretical background to illness perceptions, examine individual components of illness perceptions and look at how illness perceptions are important in understanding CFS.

Theoretical background

Illness perceptions are a relatively new area of health psychology. The field can be traced back to early work by an American health psychologist, Howard Leventhal. In the early 1980s Leventhal and his colleagues were conducting a study of lymphoma patients undergoing chemotherapy (Nerenz, Leventhal and Love 1982). Leventhal noticed that patients seemed to respond to their illness in terms of implicit theories they held about the disease and its treatment. Many patients seemed to determine the effectiveness of chemotherapy by monitoring the size of

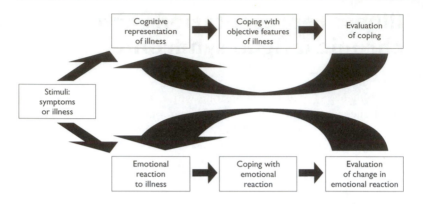

Figure 6.1 Self-regulatory model of illness behaviour.

(Adapted from Leventhal *et al.* 1984)

their palpable diseased lymph nodes. Contrary to what one might expect, patients who experienced a sudden disappearance of the nodes were more distressed than those with a gradual remission. The higher levels of distress in patients with the most rapid remission suggest that patients no longer had a useful method of assessing the effectiveness of treatment, and did not understand having to continue with a toxic treatment when they were 'cured' or had no tangible evidence of disease. The results of this study suggest patients hold an implicit model of illness in which symptoms define the presence or absence of disease and facilitate patients' psychological response.

This study and other early work led to the development of an important theoretical self-regulatory model developed by Leventhal and his colleagues (Leventhal, Meyer and Nerenz 1980; Leventhal, Nerenz and Steele 1984). This model sees illness perceptions as critical in guiding the patient's coping efforts to deal with symptoms, illness and threats to health. Leventhal and colleagues' self-regulatory model consists of four features; the cognitive representation of the illness, the emotional response to the illness and treatment, the coping directed by the illness representation and the individual's appraisal of the coping outcome (see Figure 6.1).

Research has highlighted that patients are active in trying to understand their symptoms and illness. Evidence shows that patients create illness representations which provide the basis for coping responses or procedures for dealing with threats to health (Petrie and Weinman

1997b). Consequently, when an individual experiences an unusual symptom or is provided with a diagnosis from a doctor, he or she will construct their own representation which, in turn, will determine their behaviour and other responses such as help-seeking and adherence to treatment.

The theory is easy to demonstrate with a real life example. If you experience chest pain after lunch, you may initially think it is indigestion. You may take antacid tablets and are unlikely to be worried or concerned. If, however, the pain persists and even gets worse – perhaps radiating down your arm – then there is pressure for you to revise your initial perception of the illness. Once this is done and a new cognitive model is adopted, such as 'I may be having a heart attack', then your coping strategies and emotional response are likely to be quite different.

Research using a variety of different assessment techniques suggests patients cluster their ideas about an illness around five coherent themes or components. These components together make up the patient's perception of their illness (Leventhal, Nerenz and Steele 1984). The components provide a framework for patients to make sense of their symptoms, assess health risk, and direct action and coping. Each of these components holds a perception about one aspect of the illness and together they provide the individual's coherent view of an illness.

The major cognitive components identified from research are:

- *Identity* – the label of the illness and the symptoms the patient views as being part of the disease.
- *Cause* – personal ideas about aetiology which may include simple single causes or more complex multiple causal models.
- *Time-line* – how long the patient believes the illness will last. These can be categorised into acute, chronic or episodic.
- *Consequences* – expected effects and outcome of the illness.
- *Cure-control* – how one recovers from, or controls, the illness.

These components show logical interrelationships. For example, a strong belief that the illness can be cured or controlled is typically associated with short perceived illness duration and relatively minor consequences. In contrast, beliefs that an illness will last a long time and has a number of symptoms tend to be associated with more severe consequences, perceptions and lower beliefs about cure or control of the disease.

An important question, the answer to which we know very little about at present, is where do illness beliefs come from? It is likely that as people build up knowledge and impressions of illness they develop more elaborate models of particular diseases. It is not necessary to have had direct experience with an illness. For example, we have found first-time heart attack patients to have definite ideas about the cause, controllability, time-line and consequences of their illness very soon after their admission to hospital (Petrie and Weinman 1997a). The source of people's perceptions of illness is diverse and ranges from first-hand experiences with a family member who may suffer from an illness, to information from relatives and friends as well as the media. These perceptions may lie dormant until they are activated by their own illness or that of someone close to them. As we will discuss later, with the advent of the internet more people are obtaining information from websites and patient support groups on the internet.

Patient cognitive models of their illness are, by their nature, private. Patients are often reluctant to discuss their beliefs about their illness in medical consultations because they fear being seen as stupid or misinformed. Until recently, assessment of illness perceptions has been by open-ended interviews designed to encourage patients to elaborate their own ideas of the illness. However, a questionnaire has recently been developed to measure illness perceptions in a variety of illnesses (Weinman *et al.* 1996). This questionnaire assesses perceptions on each of the five dimensions by asking patients for their own beliefs about their conditions. Examples of the items used to assess these components are shown in Table 6.1.

How illness perceptions influence coping and recovery has recently been investigated in a number of health conditions. One study has shown that patients who have suffered a recent myocardial infarction have clear beliefs about the cause, time-line, consequences and controllability of their heart condition during the acute phase of their hospital stay at a cardiac care unit. Moreover, these beliefs were associated with attendance at cardiac rehabilitation and later return to work (Petrie *et al.* 1996). This approach has now also been employed to explain responses to cancer screening (Cameron 1997), how patients cope with cancer treatment (Buick 1997), and a variety of illnesses such as diabetes (Gonder-Frederick and Cox 1991) and rheumatoid arthritis (Murphy *et al.* 1999). The next section reviews the nature of illness perceptions that are commonly found in CFS.

Table 6.1 Examples of items from the Illness Perception Questionnaire

Component	Items
Identity	Rating of a number of symptoms that the patient sees as part of the illness.
	Examples from the CFS identity scale include: nausea, sore or swollen glands, forgetfulness, dizziness, stiff or sore joints, fatigue after exercise, muscle pain.
Cause	A germ or virus caused my illness.
	Pollution of the environment caused my illness.
	Stress was a major factor in causing my illness.
Time-line	My illness is likely to be permanent rather than temporary.
	My illness will last for a long time.
Consequences	My illness has major consequences on my life.
	My illness is a serious condition.
Cure–control	There is little that can be done to improve my illness.
	What I do can determine whether my illness gets better or worse.

Illness perceptions and chronic fatigue syndrome

Identity

The identity component forms the starting point for the development of the illness representation. Typically the process begins with the experience of symptoms which triggers a search for an illness label. In Chapter 4 we showed that CFS patients often spend some time searching for a diagnosis which will both validate their suffering and provide them with a coherent picture of their illness. The interesting thing about the label of CFS is that very few people who meet diagnostic criteria for the illness actually label themselves as such (Pawlikowska *et al.* 1994). On the other hand, it is not uncommon for patients to present with a self-diagnosis of CFS who do not in fact meet criteria for the illness. A self-diagnosis of CFS is associated with higher levels of fatigue and greater psychological morbidity. This suggests that whether or not patients believe they have CFS may be a more important defining characteristic of the illness than predetermined operational criteria.

The striking feature of CFS is the large number of symptoms that sufferers associate with the illness. In a number of our studies, CFS patients endorse close to the maximum number of symptoms regardless of the length of the symptom list (Moss-Morris 1997b). The number of symptoms seen by sufferers as being part of CFS covers a far greater range than other chronic severe illnesses.

One of the consequences of associating a large number of symptoms as part of CFS is that normal symptoms may be inadvertently attributed to the illness. As we saw in Chapter 5 on symptom perception, many people report experiencing some type of symptom over a two-week period. In fact, experiencing symptoms is more common than not experiencing symptoms. Therefore it is highly likely that symptoms that may occur from time to time are mistakenly attributed to CFS and as time goes on the number of symptoms associated with the condition grows. A CFS sufferer comments on her symptoms:

> In winter I am susceptible to colds and sinus problems if I push my-self physically. In summer I have to avoid being in the sun for long as I will get very tired and get pain in my shoulder and neck.

As we have already seen, examples such as this may be consistent with Leventhal's symmetry rule (Leventhal, Meyer and Nerenz 1980) which proposes that when given a diagnostic label, an individual will seek symptoms consistent with the diagnosis. It seems likely that once the individual takes on the CFS diagnosis then a number of symptoms that occur from time to time in normal subjects are misattributed to the illness, which in turn increases the range of symptoms associated with the condition.

The other noteworthy feature of CFS patients' illness identity, discussed in Chapter 5, is the dramatic way many patients describe their symptoms. One patient told us her back feels like a Big Mac truck is leaning on it, while another described how she gets spinal whips and goes blue around the mouth when she exerts herself. A CFS patient who wrote her Master's thesis on ME described her experience as follows:

> It has been particularly difficult to write a Mastorate thesis when for six years I have never been properly awake, and never for thirty years had an instant free of pain. The irony of experiencing all 64 symptoms of ME as a participant observer and CIFID, hits me when I see notices at Massey library saying 'Study Area, Quiet Please'. There is no quiet for a student with tinnitus.

(Horne 1992:30)

Cause

Once a diagnosis of CFS has been established, from a doctor or from another source, most people spontaneously develop ideas about the cause of their illness. The process of finding a cause or causes for the illness helps individuals make sense of their illness experience and provides a framework to guide their future actions to cope with it. This is a similar process to that which occurs when individuals are confronted with an unexpected negative event such as a physical assault or accident, and indeed any serious illness (Turnquist, Harvey and Andersen 1988). Here there is also a powerful inclination to find a cause for the event (Bulman and Wortman 1977). Knowing the cause of an illness or other incident helps make the experience less anxiety-provoking and the future more predictable.

We have found on average that CFS patients attribute 70 per cent of their illness to physical causes (Moss-Morris 1997b). While they do view psychosocial factors such as stress and overwork as relevant to their illness, they see them as playing a lesser role. CFS patients are also significantly less likely to make internal psychological attributions for their illness such as 'my own behaviour' or 'my emotional state' when compared to both depressed patients and other medically ill patients (Moss-Morris 1997; Weinman *et al.* 1996). As we saw in Chapter 3, the feature of sufferers' causal models of CFS is the predominance of viral or immunological explanations for the illness. Typically, the illness is seen as being caused by an immune system that has been damaged in some way, thus allowing the entry of an unidentified virus or bacteria. The damage may occur through stress or through a reaction to allergens or pollutants. It is this immunological insult that causes the fatigue and the many other symptoms associated with CFS. This is illustrated by one CFS sufferer who comments:

> I believe that my genetic background, the environment in which I live, and the circumstances (such as heavy exposure to pesticides) have all combined to create my present condition. I believe the pesticides damaged my immune system and altered the balance of my gut flora which in turn caused me to develop food sensitivities which further suppressed my immune system so that infections are difficult for me to eradicate and also caused a rheumatic like condition to develop in my soft tissues around spine, skull, knees, and elbows.

The immunological and viral causal view of the illness is embodied in much of the information presented on CFS patient websites and newsletters. This highlights the fact that, while perceptions of illness are psychological in nature, they may be socially generated through personal contact with other sufferers or through support groups and information on the internet (Davison and Pennebaker 1997).

The internet offers support and answers for CFS sufferers but also provides a view of the illness that shapes an orthodox sufferer's view of the illness and may be intolerant of other formulations of the illness. Davison and Pennebaker (1997), in their analysis of linguistic patterns in different illness groups on the internet, comment on the view that is promoted in support groups:

> Moreover, of all the groups, CFS sufferers have the most rigidly defined boundaries about illness prototypes. This seems ironic in view of its status as a diagnosis of exclusion. Contributors' posts indicate that they are familiar with the latest research and discussions of chronic fatigue: authors who include in their writings suspected psychological factors or psychosocial treatment strategies are viewed as anathema, practically sub-human in their callous and ignorant statements ... Such intolerance reduces the information available to members, distilling and distorting, in turn, the collective illness schema.
>
> (Davison and Pennebaker 1997:479)

An example of information about the cause of CFS posted on one of the many CFS support and education groups on the internet is taken from http://www.cfs-news.org (see Table 6.2). It is interesting to analyse what the implications of these perceptions of cause may have on the way sufferers manage or cope with their CFS. The first thing to note about what is written is that it is mysterious but is generally thought to be external to the sufferer and not under the control of the patient. As well as the emotional reaction from having an illness caused by a mystery virus that attacks the immune system, this causal belief also promotes a passive stance on the part of the sufferer.

Control–cure dimension

Beliefs about the cause of CFS have a direct effect on ideas about how the illness is seen to be controlled or cured. Most CFS support groups are pessimistic about the course of the illness and the value of any treatment

Table 6.2 Internet views on the causes of CFS

What causes CFS?

The cause of the illness is not yet known. Current theories are looking at the possibilities of neuroendocrine dysfunction, viruses, environmental toxins, genetic predisposition, or a combination of these.

For a time it was thought that Epstein–Barr Virus (EBV), the cause of mononucleosis, might cause CFS but recent research has discounted this idea. The illness seems to prompt a chronic immune reaction in the body, however it is not clear that this is in response to any actual infection – this may only be a dysfunction of the immune system itself.

Some current research continues to investigate possible viral causes including HHV-6, other herpes viruses, enteroviruses, and retroviruses. Additionally, co-factors (such as genetic predisposition, stress, environment, gender, age, and prior illness) appear to play an important role in the development and course of the illness.

www.cfs-news.org

The Root Cause of CFS/FMS Is Typically 'Bad' Molecules

CFS/FMS is typically caused by 'bad' molecules that bind to good molecules inside the body and subsequently inhibit their function. Sounds simple? It is very simple conceptually. However, there are many bad and many good molecules, and tracking them is hard work.

The bad molecules are typically:

* Heavy metals such as lead, mercury, cadmium, nickel, silver, tin and barium
* Natural and synthetic chemicals and poisons (e.g. carbon monoxide, drugs)
* Pesticides (e.g. DDT)
* Natural toxins such as hydrogen sulfide, that results when fungi and bad bacteria in gut ferment sugar.
* Toxins resulting from natural waste products produced by the body that are not filtered out properly (e.g. free radicals that cause 'oxidation' of 'good' molecules).

Damage to enzymes due to bad molecules is a MAJOR issue since enzymes are used to regulate and synthesize MANY processes in the body. If a tiny bad molecule binds to a big enzyme molecule, it can take it down. Enzymes have a defense system to guard against this from occurring (e.g. thiols), yet if those defenses go down for a short period of time, the enzyme can go down, and sometimes permanently. Enzymatic damage is a BIG issue with CFS/FMS.

www.beatcfsandfms.org

beyond symptomatic relief. The New Zealand and Australia ME Society states in its information on how CFS is treated:

> Currently there is no specific treatment that cures the underlying immune system dysfunction which appears to be at the heart of the condition. Several treatments are in therapeutic trials at present. Treatment for CFS is therefore intended primarily to relieve specific symptoms.

CFS sufferers' beliefs about cure and control of the illness share similarities with how one deals with the aftermath of other viral infections (Wessely 1996b). Typically in these conditions, the symptoms cause most people to rest until they begin to feel better and their strength returns. This strong conviction in the value of rest is a pervasive theme in many CFS sufferers' views of their illness. The belief in the value of rest and a depleted immune system is illustrated in the advice of a nurse with CFS:

> Always remember, until an exciting medical announcement is made, there is no one drug to cure ME. The only cure is rest and keeping the affected parts of the body so rigid as to improve the body's defences.
>
> (Dainty 1988:49)

On the net, www.cfs-news.org advises sufferers on the best way to control CFS in its 'Frequently Asked Questions' section:

> Typically the most beneficial program is for the patient to avoid stress and to get lots of rest. This is usually the most effective regimen, among others that might also be undertaken. Stress does not merely mean unpleasant experiences, but rather any biological stressors, physical or emotional, which prompt a protective reaction in the body and which may alter physiologic equilibrium ... Failure to avoid stress often leads to short-term and long-term set-backs which may be serious. Many patients believe that if they had done more to avoid stress in the early phases of the illness, they would not have become nearly so disabled later on.

Similarly, the United Kingdom CFS site www.afme.org.uk warns CFS sufferers:

However, the low level of recognition, support and treatment means that around 60 per cent of sufferers never regain their previous level of health and up to 20 per cent become permanently disabled. If diagnosis is delayed, and sufferers are encouraged to 'push' themselves in the early stages, permanent damage can result.

The other major theme in sufferers' view of how CFS is controlled is through the use of alternative medicines and these appear in much of the advice in CFS websites. As traditional medicine is seen as having no recognised treatment for CFS it is not surprising that many patients turn to help from alternative practitioners. The CFS literature is littered with trials for alternative medicines that initially promise a great deal but usually fade from popularity only to be replaced by another new alternative possibility. Previous alternative treatments have involved high dose evening primrose oil, injections of magnesium sulphate, antihistamine and immunoglobulin therapy.

Many CFS sufferers also use antiviral agents, as well as vitamin and mineral supplements. A number of these substances are supported only by the enthusiastic claims of manufacturers keen to turn a profit. These treatments do fit with sufferers' perceptions that the illness is caused by an immune dysfunction and so many feel drawn to medicines that claim to boost their immune system and return them to full health.

Time-line and consequences dimensions

In many ways the consequences and time-line of the illness are consistent with the other illness perception components. Since the illness is typically viewed as being caused by an unidentified pathogen that attacks the immune system, and as having no immediate cure, it is not surprising that the illness course is seen as a chronic one. A smaller group of CFS sufferers, often after living with the illness for some time, endorse a cyclical view of the condition. In their case, the illness often lies dormant unless they become over-stressed or tired, when they may relapse into another extreme bout of the illness. A participant in one of our studies explained:

> The frustration caused by the unpredictability of return of symptoms is a concern. One can be feeling fine on one day and for no 'apparent' reason the next day brings forth aches, fatigue and headache.

The fact the illness is labelled *chronic* fatigue syndrome indicates that individuals perceive the course of the illness as prolonged, if not life-long. As discussed in Chapter 2, this is currently an accurate view of the illness, particularly for those CFS patients who are referred for specialist treatment. For most patients the prognosis for full recovery is poor and in follow-up studies by far the majority of cases are still disabled after 18 months, with only 2–3 per cent reporting a complete resolution of symptoms (Bombardier and Buchwald 1995; Vercoulen *et al.* 1996b).

The consequences dimension is patients' subjective view of the impact of CFS on their life. In general, illnesses that are chronic, have a large number of symptoms and have little likelihood of cure or control, are seen as having a significant impact on sufferers' lives. This is also the pattern in CFS. CFS patients have a strongly negative view of the consequences of their condition. Their perception of the consequences of the illness is greater than those held by sufferers of other chronic illnesses such as diabetes, rheumatoid arthritis and chronic pain (Weinman *et al.* 1996).

In the words of one of our research participants:

> The chronic nature of my 'fatigue' has meant that I've had time to set my lifestyle accordingly and therefore have little to compare. But it has meant a continual change of work environment which has been very disadvantageous to my own self worth and to my pocket. As a result of having no surplus energy, I have had no social life for many, many years and therefore have not developed communication skills with the kind of people who have no desire to accept or understand the problem of someone with intolerant allergies etc. I do indeed feel isolated.

For many patients, therefore, the chronic nature of their illness is inextricably linked with the devastating consequences on their lives. However, some patients do see aspects of their illness that have had more positive consequences. One CFS patient explains:

> I don't want to say it was a blessing in disguise, because that sounds horrible – 'I'm glad to get sick'. But in some ways I'm sort of glad it got me out of all those problems and really turned me around to say, 'Hey, you're not happy and you're going to have to do something to change'. I hate to say the word 'grateful', but in some ways I am.
>
> (cited in Ware 1993:67)

The positive consequences for patients appear to centre around such theses, where the illness has given them the opportunity to disengage from an unpleasant or unsatisfactory lifestyle (Ware and Kleinman 1992).

Perceptions of CFS: putting the pieces together

In studies of CFS patients we have found beliefs about the causes of the illness were notably consistent, with the majority of the patients attributing their illness to immune system dysfunction, a virus, pollution or stress. CFS patients are also less likely than other patient groups to make psychological attributions for their illness (Moss-Morris 1997b; Weinman et al. 1996). CFS patients also have particularly high scores on the identity, consequences and time-line scales, suggesting that they believe their illness has a wide range of symptoms, a profound impact on their lives and is likely to last a long time.

Unlike other groups of patients, there seems very little variation on how CFS patients view the consequences of their illness; CFS is seen as having severe effects on a wide range of life domains. Greater variation was evident on patients' views about how CFS is cured or controlled. While many sufferers are pessimistic about the effectiveness of any treatment, many see rest as an important component of any recovery.

These negative illness beliefs do demonstrate logical relationships and don't appear to be just a consequence of having a chronic physical illness. When compared to patients with rheumatoid arthritis, diabetes and chronic back pain, CFS patients had significantly higher illness identity and consequences scores (Weinman et al. 1996). Two studies found that a strong illness identity, measured by the number of symptoms patients ascribe to their illness, was associated with the beliefs that the illness is chronic, uncontrollable and has serious consequences. Time-line was also positively associated with serious consequences and negatively associated with control–cure beliefs (Heijmans 1998; Moss-Morris et al. 1996b).

Not only are illness representations distinct in CFS, but they also remain remarkably stable over time. We found that the six-month test–retest correlations for illness identity, consequences and control–cure were all greater than 0.70, while time-line had a significant correlation of 0.54 (Moss-Morris 1997). These correlations were substantially higher than those obtained from a myocardial infarction group at three and six months follow-up (Weinman et al. 1996). These findings support the cognitive behavioural formulations of CFS, which suggest that the initial belief that the illness can be cured by resting is replaced with enduring beliefs that the illness is a serious, ongoing condition which can be managed, rather than cured, by limiting activity (Surawy *et al.* 1995).

It is important to remember that illness perceptions are not restricted to the person suffering from the illness. The patient's spouse and family also have perceptions that influence the way they respond to the patient. In particular, the match between the spouse and patient in the way they believe the illness is best controlled and/or cured can have a major impact on changes to lifestyle. Spouses and family members can assist or hinder this adjustment by the degree to which they offer prompts, encouragements and other reinforcement for changes in behaviour (Weinman *et al.* in press). In a small pilot study, CFS patients who reported greater satisfaction in relationships also reported higher levels of fatigue and lower levels of activity (Schmaling and DiClementi 1995). These results suggest that supportive partners may unintentionally collude with patients in maintaining their disability. On the other hand, CFS patients whose beliefs about their illness differ from those of their spouses report less marital satisfaction, suggesting that concordance of beliefs may be important in maintaining the quality of the marital relationship (Heijmans, de Ridder and Bensing 1999).

Illness perceptions and functioning

Once an illness representation is formed it becomes a powerful force. People tend actively to process information which is consistent with their beliefs and reject inconsistent material (Gonder-Frederick and Cox 1991). Thus, people can be expected to regulate their health-related risks and to reduce health threats in a manner that is consistent with their own beliefs. CFS provides a clear example of this process. In explaining how they formulated their ideas about their illness, CFS patients describe how they relied on media reports or patient self-help groups, rather than medical advice (Clements *et al.* 1997a). These sources are more likely to confirm patients' preconceived ideas that the illness is physical and that rest is the only way to manage the condition.

Studies with CFS patients show illness perceptions to be closely associated with disability in carrying out normal daily activities. In fact, two cross-sectional studies have shown that perceptions of illness in CFS account for close to 40 per cent of the variance in self-reported disability and around 30 per cent of the variance in psychological well-being

(Heijmans and de Ridder 1998; Moss-Morris *et al.* 1996b). The component of identity and the belief in serious consequences were the most important predictors of disability. These components were also positively associated with fatigue levels, while identity was also correlated with psychological distress. On the other hand, perceptions of being personally able to control the illness were related to a greater sense of well-being.

We have also looked at whether illness representations can predict disability over time. Once again, identity was the most significant predictor of self-reported disability and fatigue levels six months later. A belief in the serious consequences of the illness was related to sickness-related unemployment and work dysfunction (Moss-Morris 1997). These results support the suggestion that illness perceptions play a role in the perpetuation of the disability in CFS.

The role of causal attributions in CFS appears to be more complex. While there is little doubt that physical attributions are a defining feature of the disorder, they are generally unrelated to ongoing disability. Cross-sectional studies of CFS patients show that neither the specific causal attributions, the number of attributions made, nor the ratio of physical to psychological attributions are associated with disability (Heijmans and de Ridder 1998; Moss-Morris 1997; Moss-Morris *et al.* 1996b). These results are consistent with two prospective primary care studies which found no relationship between specific physical attributions and the development of CFS (Cope *et al.* 1994; Wessely *et al.* 1995). Rather, the tendency to label symptoms as physical was associated with the onset of CFS following a viral infection (Cope *et al.* 1994). This suggests that the process of labelling symptoms as part of a physical disease process is more important in CFS than the actual causal attribution made. This process is similar to the concept of illness identity, which as we have already seen, is the most significant predictor of ongoing disability and distress in CFS.

Causal attributions do, however, appear to be associated with psychological adjustment and the experience of fatigue in CFS patients who have been ill for quite some time. Two studies have shown that psychological attributions for CFS are negatively associated with fatigue, but positively related to distress, while physical attributions show the opposite pattern (Heijmans and de Ridder 1998; Moss-Morris *et al.* 1996b). Attributing illness to a germ, immune system or factors such as pollution has also been shown to be protective of self-esteem, while attributions such as current stress and past trauma are associated with lower self-esteem (Moss-Morris 1997). It appears that physical attributions protect self-esteem and psychological well-being, but at the expense of fatigue levels.

In summary, CFS patients appear to have a distinct view of their illness. Their illness representation is characterised by an illness identity incorporating a broad range of symptoms. Attributions about the illness are typically external and physical, and beliefs about the chronicity and consequences of the illness are generally negative. Comparisons with other medical illness groups reveal that these negative beliefs and lack of personal responsibility for their illness are not solely a consequence of having a chronic disabling condition. The beliefs most associated with CFS-related disability are identity, or the tendency to ascribe a wide range of symptoms to the illness and a belief in the serious consequences of the illness. In the following chapter we talk about the relationship between these beliefs and coping strategies in CFS.

Chapter 7

Coping in chronic fatigue syndrome

Chronic illness poses a number of unique stresses on the individual. In the case of CFS, this stress may include the loss of life roles, coping with a range of unpleasant and confusing symptoms, dealing with medical professionals who are not always convinced about the validity of the illness, financial implications such as loss of income and ongoing medical expenses, and dealing with the emotional responses to the illness. The way in which patients cope with such stress can determine how well they adapt to their illness, and in some cases, whether or not they recover from it. Adaptation to the illness can be defined as both the level of disability afforded by the illness and the psychological responses to it.

The self-regulatory model presented in the previous chapter provides a theoretical framework for understanding coping in CFS. The way in which patients conceptualise their illness is seen to drive their coping responses. The ability of these responses to reduce the stresses associated with the illness are then appraised, and if needs be, the responses are modified. The cognitive behavioural model of CFS discussed in Chapter 4 provides an illustration of how this process may occur both in the early and later stages of the illness (Surawy *et al.* 1995).

In the development phase, the way in which patients cope may be important in the progression to CFS. Some patients may try to rush back to their pre-illness levels of activity too early. This in itself produces symptoms which may then be appraised by the patient as signs of continuing disease. The coping response may then be to rest and reduce levels of activity. Resting reduces the symptoms and so once again the patient rushes back to previous commitments. Once this cycle is repeated the patient begins to observe that bursts of activity are unhelpful responses to the illness. On the other hand, resting reduces symptoms so the belief develops that this is the best way to deal with the illness. This causes patients to monitor their bodies vigilantly for signs of illness and to reduce activity levels accordingly.

In this chapter we begin by looking at the different ways in which patients deal with their CFS and how these different strategies are related to both illness beliefs and adaptative outcome. While limiting activity is one of the key coping strategies used by CFS patients, as will be seen from this discussion, a number of other strategies are also important. In the final section, we discuss treatment approaches aimed at helping CFS patients to cope better with their illness.

Coping by limiting activity

Most CFS patients believe that rest and reduced activity is helpful in controlling symptoms, while maintaining activity is unhelpful (Ray, Jefferies and Weir 1995). This limiting coping style, distinguishes CFS patients from depressed patients, suggests that this form of coping may be one of the defining features of the illness (Moss-Morris 1997).

An interesting pattern emerges from patients' accounts of how they limit their activity. Rather than consistently limiting activity, they adjust their levels depending on how they are feeling at any one time. One patient explains:

> I lead an active life but need to rest for some time each day. It may be as little as half an hour, depending on what stage of illness I'm at. If I get really exhausted or am having a bad relapse, I will go to bed for a day or two if possible. This is contrary to what I was earlier advised, but it works well for me … I know I will go downhill if I don't stop and rest. I therefore make it a priority wherever possible.
>
> (Frazer 1995:18)

Another patient describes how she runs her business at home, so that she can accommodate her work demands around her illness:

> I could never hold a job outside. Because of the flexibility. If I'm sick, I can rest. When my energy is low, like during the day, I can take it easy, then work until 11.00 at night.
>
> (cited in Ware 1998:399)

In accommodating to the illness CFS patients have to organise and plan their lives in order to avoid over-exertion, and they also have to control their stress levels (Ray *et al.* 1993b). As one CFS patient told us:

> One becomes very self protective and avoids where possible likely stressful situations both physical and emotional.

We have found that CFS patients who limit activity and stress also tend to restrict their dietary and alcohol intake. Each patient seems to develop his or her own beliefs around which foods should be avoided and the self-help literature is inundated with such narratives:

> Elimination of caffeine and dairy products has reduced discomfort in the muscles, particularly the throat area. When in the past muscular discomfort has been present and increases, it is a sign for me to slow down and reserve energy.
>
> I restrict my exposure to chemicals as much as possible (that is, no perfumes, detergents, cleaning fluids, etc). This is also an important tool for me. My diet, although not as restricted as it used to be, is still very limited ... I basically follow a plain diet with little strong flavourings or chemical additives, as well as little or no alcohol.
>
> (Frazer 1995:18)

Limiting activity, illness beliefs and adjustment

The behavioural responses of limiting activity and stress are associated with patients' beliefs that resting is a helpful way of controlling symptoms (Ray *et al.* 1995). Similarly, a sense of personal control over the illness is positively associated with limiting activity (Moss-Morris 1997). Thus, for CFS patients limiting activity appears to be a way of controlling the illness. Limiting activity is also related to a more positive outlook on the illness. CFS patients who have a very negative view of the consequences and time-line of their illness are less likely to use limiting activity than those who do not. For some patients these strategies are also seen as an eventual cure. One patient explains:

> I have been through trauma in my attitude to my illness, but I am now accepting of it and in fact feel calm and serene. While not seeing it as

a lifetime sentence I feel that rest and not accepting tasks or putting myself in stressful situations is the best cure.

Limiting activity and stress has a particularly interesting relationship to disability in CFS. As would be predicted, both longitudinal and cross-sectional results have shown that limiting strategies result in higher levels of dysfunction (Moss-Morris 1997; Ray, Jefferies and Weir 1997; Ray *et al.* 1995; Sharpe *et al.* 1992). One longitudinal study found that this was particularly true for patients who had been ill for longer periods of time, suggesting that as time goes by, the more one limits activity and stress, the less one feels able to do (Ray *et al.* 1997). Another longitudinal study found that work was particularly affected. Limiting activity strategies predicted fewer working hours per week, a decreased likelihood of increasing work hours, and higher levels of self-reported disruption to work six months later (Moss-Morris 1997).

These same strategies are also related to feelings of positive well-being (Moss-Morris 1997). At first glance these findings appear contradictory: surely a decreased capacity to work and participate in day-to-day activities would lead to feelings of demoralization and distress? However, as discussed above, limiting strategies may provide CFS patients with a sense of control over the illness and a feeling that they are actively doing something to deal with the problem. Decreasing activity and stress levels could also help to temper symptoms and reduce the distress of illness unpredictability (Ray *et al.* 1997). Further, believing they need to accommodate to the illness may provide people with a legitimate reason to remove themselves from situations they had previously found stressful.

There is also some evidence that limiting activity may be related to the onset of CFS. Two prospective studies of patients following viral infections found that prolonged convalescence or doctor-sanctioned time off work were predictors of the development of chronic fatigue (Cope *et al.* 1994; Hotopf, Noah and Wessely 1996). While these results are obviously not conclusive, they suggest that prolonged periods of inactivity may be unhelpful in the early stages of the illness.

Maintaining activity

Although most CFS patients believe that maintaining activity is harmful to their illness, there are a small group of patients who report pushing themselves to stay active regardless of how it affects their symptoms

(Ray *et al.* 1995; Ray *et al.* 1993b). Self-reports suggest that this coping style may be more common in the earlier stages of the illness. A 32-year-old student nurse describes:

> I was advised that, following this illness, recurrences are common and they should disappear in time. I still believed this when I started training as a nurse. I enjoyed the training immensely, and expected to feel more tired than the other students on account of my age and the fact that I had a home to run. I did well in my training, and worked and studied hard, but after a while the gruelling life began to take its toll of my health. My relapses became more frequent and, in my ignorance, I tried to battle on.
>
> (N.P. cited in Wookey 1986:87)

For others, maintaining activity appears to be related to a sense of necessity. One student with CFS explains that she is able to continue with her studies, but does not believe she will get better until she stops working for a while:

> After my studies are completed I plan to go on the sickness benefit or 'live off my parents' in a serious bid to get better as soon as possible. I don't want to stay sick but up until now I have given my studies priority over my health.

Maintaining activity appears to reduce functional impairment in CFS but there is also some evidence that it is related to higher anxiety levels (Ray *et al.* 1995; Ray *et al.* 1993b). The higher anxiety levels may reflect the fact that most patients believe that maintaining activity is harmful to their illness, and that in many cases, pushing to keep going is seen as a necessity rather than a helpful coping strategy.

Focussing on symptoms and disengagement

Interviews with CFS patients have identified another key coping strategy, focussing on symptoms (Ray *et al.* 1993b). This reflects a preoccupation with symptoms and a feeling of helplessness in the face of the illness. Two patients provide vivid descriptions of this process:

> After suffering the debilitating effects of ME/CFS I know how crucial it is to listen to your body and in no way should one push oneself

beyond one's physical state as the result is very likely to put one back into relapse and take even longer to recover. This is *not* just tiredness but a profound weakness which words cannot describe, and is so incapacitating one can virtually do nothing to fight back. One can only wait until the extreme weakness has lifted.

When I'm in a relapse I just can't cope and resent the fact that I have ME, but I worry in between relapses that perhaps I have something more serious that doctors haven't found – as I feel so utterly ill and tired most or all of the time. Sometimes I get tired of being ill and wish I could die, because I feel so awful.

Focussing on symptoms seems to be closely related to a coping strategy identified in the general coping literature called disengagement. Disengagement is the process of giving up in the face of a stressor that appears to be overwhelming. Studies on patients with a range of chronic illnesses have shown that disengagement strategies are consistently related to poor adaptation (Petrie and Moss-Morris 1997). Similarly, disengagement strategies in CFS have shown consistent relationships to disability, fatigue and psychological distress (Antoni *et al.* 1994; Heijmans 1998; Moss-Morris *et al.* 1996b; Ray *et al.* 1997; Ray *et al.* 1995).

Not only are disengagement coping strategies particularly maladaptive, but they also seem to distinguish CFS patients from others. Blakely and colleagues (1991) compared coping in CFS patients, chronic pain patients and healthy controls. The CFS group were significantly more likely than the others to use disengagement strategies in dealing with stressful situations.

Disengagement strategies are also associated with more negative illness beliefs. CFS patients' beliefs about illness identity, serious consequences, and chronic time-line were positively associated with both disengagement strategies and focussing on symptoms, while a sense of internal control over the illness was negatively related (Heijmans 1998; Moss-Morris 1997; Moss-Morris *et al.* 1996b). Interestingly, disengagement was also associated with emotional rather than physical attributions for the illness. These results confirm that disengaging from dealing with the CFS is a conceptually different coping strategy to limiting activity and stress. We have already seen that limiting strategies are associated with positive illness beliefs and a greater sense of well-being.

Information seeking

It is obvious from the self-help literature on CFS that patients are constantly on the lookout for new information which confirms the validity of their illness. Patients are often very well informed of the latest research developments, particularly studies which investigate the biological concomitants of the illness. In many cases, patients feel that they know more about their CFS than their doctors:

> I have so much knowledge, you know, that I would like to be able to share. Just from sort of observing people's stories ... I probably know more than the average GP about the cause of the illness.
>
> (cited in Ax *et al.* 1997:251)

This information seeking is also reflected in a readiness to try new remedies for the illness:

> I have tried many treatments and 'cures' over the years. These have included homeopathy, naturopathy, vitamins, magnesium, vitamin B12 injections, Transfer Factor Gamma Globulin, cold water bath therapy, psychiatry, self-analysis, and various exercise programmes. Some of these treatments have been beneficial, while others have had limited benefits. I still, however, find the neuro-cognitive symptoms the most disturbing and difficult to manage. So if anyone has any brilliant ideas, please let me know!
>
> (Frazer 1995:18)

A longitudinal study found that patients who reported high levels of information seeking at initial assessment reported significantly higher levels of fatigue one year later. This way of coping may reflect or give rise to an exacerbated concern about symptoms. Alternatively, constantly seeking information which does not lead to the expected solutions may increase the fatigue experienced over time.

Positive reinterpretation and seeking social support

Two coping strategies, positive reinterpretation (finding something positive in the situation) and seeking support for emotional reasons, are consistently related to psychological adjustment to chronic illnesses (Petrie and Moss-Morris 1997). Interviews with CFS patients confirm that a number of patients report making substantial lifestyle changes as the result of their illness. For many these changes were viewed positively. Patients expressed the new-found ability to take care of their own needs rather than those of others, and to value feelings of contentment over those of success (Ware 1993; Ware and Kleinman 1992). A CFS patient explains:

> I've lost a lot, but I've gained more than I've lost. I think in the beginning I lost self-respect. I lost a lot of things. I felt abandoned. I was frightened. It's been a very frightening experience but I am a better person for it. Not worse, no. Much better.
>
> (cited in Ware 1993:68)

Other patients talk about the importance of social support in relation to their illness:

> I find the biggest factor that got me through CFS, is the support I got from my husband and my family. Being around positive people, and people who understood the illness, is part of the therapy.

CFS patients who believe they have some control over their illness are more likely to use positive reinterpretation as a coping strategy (Moss-Morris *et al.* 1996b). In turn, positive reinterpretation is related to a greater sense of psychological well-being. Seeking emotional social support is related to lower levels of disability and greater psychological adjustment to the illness. There is also some evidence that positive reinterpretation protects against the development of CFS. A nested case–control study of patients presenting to a general practice with either a viral infection or general complaint found that those who reported using cognitive coping were less likely to develop CFS six months later (Chalder *et al.*, in submission).

Coping pathways in CFS

In general, the findings suggest that two disparate pathways of illness perceptions, coping and disability may exist. CFS patients who hold excessively negative beliefs tend to give up or withdraw from dealing with the illness and focus excessively on their symptoms. Rather than actively choosing to limit their activity, their negative illness beliefs may lead to feelings of helplessness and loss of control, resulting in a passive withdrawal from activity and heightened negative effects. On the other side is the group of patients with less pessimistic illness beliefs, who nevertheless experience a number of symptoms which they strongly attribute to signs of a physical disease. These patients believe that rest is the effective way of dealing with their symptoms, and as a result choose to limit their exposure to stress and activity. They feel more in control of their illness and are psychologically better adjusted to their condition, but are still unduly disabled.

In addition to these key coping strategies there is also individual variation in the use of other adaptive strategies such as seeking social support and positive reinterpretation, as well as less adaptive strategies, such as information seeking. It is still unclear at this stage how these strategies are used in combination, and how various combinations of strategies may influence outcome.

Taken together, the results from studies which have investigated coping in CFS provide additional support for the heterogeneous nature of CFS. The current cognitive behavioural models of CFS do not take into account the possibility that different cognitive behavioural profiles may lead to the same symptom presentation, but different degrees of disability. The current models focus mostly on the active decision to limit activity rather than the passive withdrawal from dealing with the problem. This distinction is important as it may have implications for cognitive behavioural treatment.

Coping treatments for chronic fatigue syndrome

Two therapeutic approaches have been used to increase the quality of life of CFS patients. The first is cognitive behavioural therapy. This approach aims to show patients that activity can be steadily and safely increased without exacerbating symptoms. The graded return to activity is presented in conjunction with techniques to challenge and alter maladaptive thought patterns. The treatment itself is collaborative and negotiated with the patient. A schedule of planned, graded activity and rest is initially agreed upon. Patients are encouraged to keep their initial targets modest, and small enough to be sustained despite fluctuations in symptoms. Activity and rest are pre-planned and consistent rather than symptom-driven. Patients are encouraged to persevere with their targets, and not to reduce them on a bad day, nor exceed them on a good day.

Cognitive strategies are introduced while the graded activity programme continues. The aim of these strategies is to develop thinking patterns which promote recovery. Patients are asked to record any unhelpful or distressing thoughts and to practise generating less catastrophic, more helpful alternatives. The focus is on re-evaluating the meaning and consequences of symptoms as well as addressing issues such as perfectionism, self-criticism, guilt and performance expectations.

Graded exercise programmes focus largely on slowly increasing exercise levels. Patients are also encouraged to set weekly goals and to increase their exercise in accordance with these goals rather than their symptoms. Once again, the approach is collaborative and patients are encouraged to start by setting goals that are easily manageable. Patients are also encouraged not to exceed their target exercise. In the following sections, we review the results from randomised controlled trials which have used these approaches with CFS patients.

Cognitive behavioural therapy for chronic fatigue syndrome

Cognitive behaviour therapy focuses on changing the beliefs patients hold about their illness and their ideas about the most effective ways to manage the illness. Five cognitive behavioural therapy (CBT) trials with CFS patients have been completed. Of these, two reported that CBT was no more effective than standard medical care, immunological treatment (Friedberg and Krupp 1994; Lloyd et al. 1993) or no treatment, while three others found that CBT was significantly more effective than relaxation therapy (Deale et al. 1997), standard medical care (Sharpe et al. 1996b) and no treatment (Butler et al. 1991). The conflicting results most likely reflect the different approaches used in the individual trials. The successful trials could be distinguished from the non-successful ones in that they were based on a gradual return to activity with gentle challenging of patients' existing illness beliefs.

CFS patients in these successful CBT trials reported substantial and continued improvement in their general functioning, levels of fatigue and depression up to a year post-treatment, although few reported complete resolution of symptoms (Butler et al. 1991; Deale et al. 1997; Sharpe et al. 1996b). A four-year follow-up of the first successful CBT trial showed that patients who initially responded to treatment sustained their level of functional improvement, while those who initially refused or did not benefit from treatment were still substantially disabled by their CFS (Bonner *et al.* 1994). Deale and colleagues (1998) demonstrated that changes in the beliefs about the harmful effects of activity were predictive of improvement following CBT while changes in causal attributions were not, providing support for the idea that this is a key ingredient in this therapeutic approach.

One of the unsuccessful CBT trials also included graded activity as part of the treatment, but failed to address illness or symptom beliefs (Lloyd *et al.* 1993). In fact, as they combined their CBT trial with an immunological trial, the concurrent administration of immunoglobin injections may even have confirmed patients' beliefs about the essentially physical nature of the illness. The number of CBT sessions included in this trial may also have been too few to bring about significant change. The rationale behind Friedberg and Krupp's (1994) CBT trial was distinctly different from the successful trials. Rather than challenging existing illness beliefs and increasing activity, patients were encouraged to accept their symptoms, to tolerate illness limitations, and to restructure their lifestyle in keeping with the confines imposed by the illness. Although this programme had some effect on depressive symptoms, there were no significant changes in stress symptoms or fatigue severity. Overall it appears that for CBT to be effective, beliefs about the illness must be addressed.

Two of the successful CBT trials were well designed randomised controlled trials (Deale *et al.* 1997; Sharpe *et al.* 1996b). When compared to results from other CFS treatment trials, the effects of cognitive behavioural therapy are quite substantial (Wessely 1996b). Nevertheless, there is a marked backlash against this form of therapy in the CFS self-help literature. A recent editorial in a local ME magazine provided a summary of cognitive behavioural theories of CFS and provided the following commentary on the effectiveness of the therapy:

> This is achieved by applying this school's particular form of CBT. This means a) convincing the patient that they have not got a physical illness and b) administering a graded exercise programme. This consists of continually but gradually increasing aerobic exercise in which allowances are not made for patient relapses. Their trials claim to show that this form of CBT is effective in curing 80 per cent of sufferers and therefore indirectly helps prove their theory is correct. This however is not a direct cause effect relationship. To me it appears to be difficult to 'prove' a psychological theory by research

and therefore this indirect approach remains acceptable. This is like saying if broken legs can be fixed with plaster casts then the initial cause of the bone problem is lack of plaster!

(Booth 1998:11)

One of the major drawbacks, therefore, of CBT is its lack of acceptability to patients. This means only a small percentage of patients may ever present for this form of treatment. Further, while the successful trials have shown substantial improvements, few patients report a complete recovery and a small percentage do not improve. More work is needed to determine who benefits from CBT. The fact that different coping styles and beliefs may lead to CFS suggests that future programmes should be tailored according to these individual needs.

Graded exercise for chronic fatigue syndrome

The results from two trials of graded exercise for CFS have shown promising results. A twelve-week randomised trial of graded exercise which used physical flexibility training as a placebo control showed that graded exercise significantly improved physical functioning and reduced fatigue levels (Fulcher and White 1997). This trial used the approach outlined at the beginning of this section. The level at which patients should be exercising was based on their current levels of fitness and was prescribed by an exercise physiologist. Patients were given heart rate monitors so that they could ensure that they met, but did not exceed, their target heart rate. This provided patients with an external device to monitor their physical state, rather than monitoring how much they should do by focussing on their symptoms. A key finding from this trial was that the objective measures of physical fitness were not associated with clinical improvement. This suggests that the success of this approach may lie in altering patients' fears about activity and exercise.

Another study, which compared fluoxetine or placebo in combination with exercise or no exercise, also found that patients undergoing exercise treatment showed significant improvements in physical functioning and fatigue (Wearden et al. 1998). While the drop-out rate from this trial was higher than the previous trial, possibly due to the fact that the graded exercise was less structured and prescriptive, the positive results for exercise were maintained even when the drop-out rate was taken into consideration.

Interestingly, although most CFS patients appear to avoid exercise, there are examples in the self-help literature of patients who intuitively use this graded exercise approach to deal with their symptoms:

> I decided I would channel all my energy into doing as much as I could every day. I knew that I would have my bad days but I was determined that I would not let the bad days get me down. I decided that I would respect my illness and rest when I was forced to, but at the same time try to live as normal a life as possible ... I started doing a gentle exercise program and although I found it induced fatigue, my recovery time improved. As I managed to exercise and work harder, my confidence grew. There was always the fear in the background that overactivity would induce a relapse and I was never sure how far to push my body. Despite the fear, I kept pushing through barriers, some associated with a lot of pain especially in the legs. At present I see more than 110 patients a week. I am up at 6.00 a.m. every morning ...
>
> (Lopis 1995:16)

> I worked in gradual increments over a two-year time span. For me, it was a major fact in my recovery. I don't mean to lay a guilt trip on anybody by saying I regularly jog two miles. But if I don't say anything about it, it would be like withholding the name of a medication or supplement that had given me great improvement.
>
> (Dopperpuhl 1998:37)

> This is my second year activity running, tramping, cycling and skiing after almost 5 years of very little exercise. The come-back was not easy. It was a case of a little bit at a time and knowing when to stop and rest. I can still tire easily, but if I stop in time and avoid stress, then I bounce back very quickly ... it is a case of slowly setting goals and taking positive control of your body, mind and soul.
>
> (Greg 1991–1992:35)

The theme in each of these accounts is that it was a slow, gradual process. Overcoming fear of activity also seems to be an important ingredient. These narratives are different to the accounts where patients talk about maintaining activity. Here, patients seem to believe that exercise is helpful, whereas CFS patients who maintain activity often do not.

It is worth noting that neither CBT nor graded exercise treatment seem to have much impact on patients' moods. This is an important area for future investigation as CFS patients are generally more distressed than other groups of medically ill patients. Nevertheless, these appear to be promising treatments for CFS. These approaches have the advantage of offering assistance to patients regardless of the cause of the illness, as they focus on perpetuating rather than precipitating factors. Similar approaches are used with a wide range of other medical illnesses as well as psychological disorders. Thus, the argument of whether the illness is physical or psychological can largely be avoided. The success of the treatment appears to be more closely related to changes in the beliefs about the harmful effects of activity, rather than changes in beliefs about the cause of the illness.

In summary, we feel that the information reviewed in this book suggests that it is unlikely that a simple cause and treatment will ever be found for CFS. It appears to be a multifactorial heterogenous illness. At this stage, approaches which assist patients to decrease their levels of disability appear to be promising. More work is needed to investigate why the approaches are not successful for all patients and how the approaches can be optimised. It may be that graded exercise is a better treatment for some patients, while cognitive behavioural therapy works better for others. Assisting patients to minimise their distress also needs to be addressed in future treatment approaches.

References

Abbey, S. E. (1996) 'Psychiatric diagnostic overlap in chronic fatigue syndrome', in M. A. Demitrack and S. E. Abbey (eds), *Chronic Fatigue Syndrome: An Integrated Approach to Evaluation and Treatment*, New York: Guilford Press.

Abbey, S. E. and Garfinkel, P. E. (1991) 'Chronic fatigue syndrome and depression: cause, effect, or covariate', *Reviews of Infectious Diseases*, 13(Suppl. 1), S73–83.

Ablashi, D. V. (1994) 'Viral studies of chronic fatigue syndrome', *Clinical Infectious Diseases* 18(Suppl. 1), S130–3.

Allain, T. J., Bearn, J. A., Coskeran, P., Jones, J., Checkley, A., Butler, J., Wessely, S. and Miell, J. P. (1997) 'Changes in growth hormone, insulin, insulin-like growth factors (IGFs), and IGF-binding protein-1 in chronic fatigue syndrome', *Biological Psychiatry*, 41(5), 567–73.

Altay, H. T., Toner, B. B., Brooker, H., Abbey, S. E., Salit, I. E. and Garfinkel, P. E. (1990) 'The neuropsychological dimensions of post-infectious neuromyasthenia (chronic fatigue syndrome): a preliminary report', *International Journal of Psychiatry in Medicine* 20(2), 141–9.

Anderson, J. S. and Estwing Ferrans, C. (1997) 'The quality of life of persons with chronic fatigue syndrome', *Journal of Nervous and Mental Disease* 185, 359–67.

Anonymous (1956) 'A new clinical entity?' (editorial), *Lancet* 26, 789–90.

Antoni, M. H., Brickman, A., Lutgendorf, S., Klimas, N., Imia-Fins, A., Ironson, G., Quillian, R., Miguez, M. J., van Riel, F., Morgan, R., Patarca, R. and Fletcher M. A. (1994) 'Psychosocial correlates of illness burden in chronic fatigue syndrome', *Clinical Infectious Diseases* 18(Suppl. 1), S73–8.

Ax, S., Greg, V. H. and Jones, D. (1997) 'Chronic fatigue syndrome: sufferers' evaluation of medical support', *Journal of the Royal Society of Medicine* 90, 250–24.

Bakheit, A. M., Behan, P. O., Dinan, T. G., Gray, C. E. and Keane, V. (1992)

'Possible upregulation of hypothalamic 5-hydroxytryptamine receptors in patients with post-viral fatigue syndrome', *British Medical Journal* 304, 1010–12.

Bakheit, A. M., Behan, P. O., Watson, W. S. and Morton, J. J. (1993) 'Abnormal arginine vasopressin secretion and water metabolism in patients with postviral fatigue syndrome', *Acta Neurologica Scandinavia* 87, 234–8.

Barsky, A. J. and Borus, J. F. (1999) 'Functional Somatic Syndromes', *Annals of Internal Medicine* 130, 910–21.

Bates, D. W., Buchwald, D., Lee, J., Kith, P., Doolittle, T., Rutherford, C., Churchill, W. H., Schur, P. H., Wener, M., Wybenga, D., Winkelman, J. and Komaroff, A. L. (1995) 'Clinical laboratory test findings in patients with chronic fatigue syndrome', *Archives of Internal Medicine* 155(1), 97–103.

Bates, D. W., Buchwald, D., Lee, J., Kith, P., Doolittle, T. H., Umali, P. and Komaroff, A. L. (1994) 'A comparison of case definitions of chronic fatigue syndrome', *Clinical Infectious Diseases* 18(Suppl. 1), S11–5.

Bates, D. W., Schmitt, W., Buchwald, D., Ware, N. C., Lee, J., Thoyer, E., Kornish, R. J. and Komaroff, A. L. (1993) 'Prevalence of fatigue and chronic fatigue syndrome in a primary care practice', *Archives of Internal Medicine* 153(24), 2759–65.

Bazelmans, E., Bleijenberg, G., Vercoulen, J., Vandermeer, J. W. M. and Folgering, H. (1997) 'The Chronic Fatigue Syndrome and Hyperventilation', *Journal of Psychosomatic Research* 43(4), 371–7.

Beard, G. (1869) 'Neurasthenia or nervous exhaustion', *Boston Medical and Surgical Journal* 3, 217–20.

Bearn, J., Allain, T., Coskeran, P., Munro, N., Butler, J., McGregor, A. and Wessely, S. (1995) 'Neuroendocrine responses to d-fenfluramine and insulin-induced hypoglycemia in chronic fatigue syndrome', *Biological Psychiatry* 37(4), 245–52.

Bearn, J. and Wessely, S. (1994) 'Neurobiological aspects of the chronic fatigue syndrome', *European Journal of Clinical Investigation* 24(2), 79–90.

Bennett, A. L., Fagioli, L. R., Schur, P. H., Schacterle, R. S. and Komaroff, A. L. (1996) 'Immunoglobin subclass levels in chronic fatigue syndrome', *Journal of Clinical Immunology* 16, 315–20.

Berelowitz, G. J., Burgess, A. P., Thanabalasingham, T., Murray-Lyon, I. M. and Wright, D. J. (1995) 'Post-hepatitis syndrome revisited', *Journal of Viral Hepatitis* 2(3), 133–8.

Blakely, A. A., Howard, R. C., Sosich, R. M., Murdoch, J. C., Menkes, D. B. and Spears, G. F. S. (1991) 'Psychiatric symptoms, personality and ways of coping in chronic fatigue syndrome', *Psychological Medicine* 21, 347–62.

Bloom, J. R. and Monterossa, S. (1981) 'Hypertension labeling and sense of well-being', *American Journal of Public Health* 71, 1228–32.

Bombardier, C. H. and Buchwald, D. (1995) 'Outcome and prognosis in patients with chronic fatigue and chronic fatigue syndrome', *Archives of Internal Medicine* 155, 2105–10.

Bonner, D., Ron, M., Chalder, T., Butler, S. and Wessely, S. (1994) 'Chronic fatigue syndrome: a follow up study', *Journal of Neurology, Neurosurgery and Psychiatry* 57(5), 617–21.

Booth, J. (1996) Editorial, *Meeting-Place* 48, 2.

Booth, J. (1998) 'Dr Simon Wessely: Prophet or profit?', *Meeting-Place* Spring, 9–13.

Booth, J. (1999a) 'Understanding the emotional rollercoaster in CFS', *Meeting-Place* 57, 35.

Booth, J. (1999b) 'Neuroendocrine disturbances', *Meeting-Place* 57, 17.

Bou-Holaigah, I., Rowe, P. C., Kan, J. and Calkins, H. (1995) 'The relationship between neurally mediated hypotension and the chronic fatigue syndrome', *Journal of the American Medical Association* 274(12), 961–7.

Briggs, N. C. and Levine, P. H. (1994) 'A comparative review of systematic and neurological symptomatology in 12 outbreaks collectively described as chronic fatigue syndrome, epidemic neuromyasthenia, and myalgic encephalomyelitis', *Clinical Infectious Diseases* 18(Suppl. 1), S32– S42.

Broom, D. H. and Woodward, R. V. (1996) 'Medicalisation reconsidered: toward a collaborative approach to care', *Sociology of Health and Illness* 18, 357–78.

Bruce-Jones, W. D., White, P. D., Thomas, J. M. and Clare, A. W. (1994) 'The effect of social adversity on the fatigue syndrome, psychiatric disorders and physical recovery, following glandular fever', *Psychological Medicine* 24(3), 651–9.

Buchwald, D. (1996) 'Fibromyalgia and chronic fatigue syndrome: similarities and differences', *Rheumatic Diseases Clinics of North America* 22(2), 219–43.

Buchwald, D., Ashley, R. L., Pearlman, T., Kith, P. and Komaroff, A. L. (1996) 'Viral serologies in patients with chronic fatigue and chronic fatigue syndrome', *Journal of Medical Virology* 50(1), 25–30.

Buchwald, D., Cheney, P. R., Peterson, D. L., Henry, B., Wormsley, S. B., Geiger, A., Ablashi, D. V., Salahuddin, S. Z., Saxinger, C., Biddle, R., Kikinis, R., Jolesz, F. F., Folks, T., Balachandran, N., Peter, J. B., Gallo, R. C. and Komaroff, A. L. (1992) 'A chronic illness characterized by fatigue, neurologic and immunologic disorders, and active human herpes virus type 6 infection', *Annals of Internal Medicine* 116(2), 103–13.

Buchwald, D. and Garrity, D. (1994) 'Comparison of patients with chronic fatigue syndrome, fibromyalgia, and multiple chemical sensitivities', *Archives of Internal Medicine* 154(18), 2049–53.

Buchwald, D., Goldenberg, D. L., Sullivan, J. L. and Komaroff, A. L. (1987)

'The "chronic, active Epstein–Barr virus infection" syndrome and primary fibromyalgia', *Arthritis and Rheumatism* 30, 1132–6.

Buchwald, D. and Komaroff, A. L. (1991) 'Review of laboratory findings for patients with chronic fatigue syndrome', *Reviews of Infectious Diseases* 13(Suppl. 1), S12–18.

Buckley, L., MacHale, S. M., Cavanagh, J. T., Sharpe, M., Deary, I. J. and Lawrie, S. M. (1999) 'Personality dimensions in chronic fatigue syndrome and depression', *Journal of Psychosomatic Research* 46(4), 395–400.

Buick, D. L. (1997) 'Illness representations and breast cancer: coping with radiation and chemotherapy', in K. J. Petrie and J. Weinman (eds), *Perceptions of Health and Illness*, London: Harwood Academic.

Bulman, J. R. and Wortman, C. B. (1977) 'Attributions of blame and coping in the 'real world': severe accident victims react to their lot', *Journal of Personality and Social Psychology* 35, 351–63.

Butler, S., Chalder, T., Ron, M. and Wessely, S. (1991) 'Cognitive behaviour therapy in chronic fatigue syndrome', *Journal of Neurology, Neurosurgery and Psychiatry* 54(2), 153–8.

Cameron, L. D. (1997) 'Screening for cancer: illness perception and illness worry', in K. J. Petrie and J. Weinman (eds), *Perceptions of Health and Illness*, London: Harwood Academic.

Cameron, R. S. (1995) 'The cost of long term disability due to fibromyalgia, chronic fatigue syndrome and repetitive strain injury: the private insurance perspective', *Journal of Musculoskeletal Pain* 3, 169–72.

Cathebras, P., Robbins, J., Kirmayer, L. and Hayton, B. (1992) 'Fatigue in primary care: prevalence, psychiatric co-morbidity, illness behaviour and outcome', *Journal of General Internal Medicine* 7, 278–86.

Chalder, T., Neeleman, J., Power, M. and Wessely, S. (in submission) 'The role of life events, social support and coping in chronic fatigue'.

Clark, M. R., Katon, W., Russo, J., Kith, P., Sintay, M. and Buchwald, D. (1995) 'Chronic fatigue: risk factors for symptom persistence in a 2½-year follow-up study', *American Journal of Medicine* 98(2), 187–95.

Cleare, A. J., Bearn, J., Allain, T., McGregor, A., Wessely, S., Murray, R. M. and O'Keane, V. (1995) 'Contrasting neuroendocrine responses in depression and chronic fatigue syndrome', *Journal of Affective Disorders* 34(4), 283–9.

Cleare, A. J., Heap, E., Malhi, G. S., Wessely, S., O'Keane, V. and Miell, J. (1999) 'Low-dose hydrocortisone in chronic fatigue syndrome: a randomised crossover trial', *Lancet* 353(9151), 455–8.

Clements, A., Sharpe, M., Simkin, S., Borrill, J. and Hawton, K. (1997a) 'Chronic fatigue syndrome: a qualitative investigation of patients' beliefs about the illness', *Journal of Psychosomatic Research* 42(6), 615–24.

Clements, A., Sharpe, M., Simkin, S., Borrill, J. and Hawton, K. (1997b) 'Illness beliefs of patients with chronic fatigue syndrome: a qualitative investigation', *Journal of Psychosomatic Research* 42, 615–24.

Conti, F., Magrini, L., Priori, R., Valesini, G. and Bonini, S. (1996) 'Eosinophil cationic protein serum levels and allergy in chronic fatigue syndrome', *Allergy* 51, 124–7.

Cooper, L. (1997) 'Myalgic encephalomyelitis and the medical encounter', *Sociology of Health and Illness* 19, 186–207.

Cope, H., David, A., Pelosi, A. and Mann, A. (1994) 'Predictors of chronic "postviral" fatigue', *Lancet* 344, 864–8.

Cope, H. and David, A. S. (1996) 'Neuroimaging in chronic fatigue syndrome' (editorial), *Journal of Neurology, Neurosurgery and Psychiatry* 60(5), 471–3.

Cope, H., Mann, A., Pelosi, A. and David, A. (1996) 'Psychosocial risk factors for chronic fatigue and chronic fatigue syndrome following presumed viral illness: a case–control study', *Psychological Medicine* 26(6), 1197–209.

Cope, H., Pernet, A., Kendall, B. and David, A. (1995) 'Cognitive functioning and magnetic resonance imaging in chronic fatigue', *British Journal of Psychiatry* 167(1), 86–94.

Costa, P. T., McCrae, R. R., Zonderman, A. B., Barbano, H. E., Lebowitz, B. and Larson, D. M. (1986) 'Cross-sectional studies of personality in a national sample: 2. Stability in neuroticism, extraversion and openness', *Psychology and Aging* 1, 144–9.

Crashley, S. (1997) 'Tilting table creates CFS horror and hope', *New Zealand Doctor* 22 January, 36.

Croyle, R. T. and Sande, G. N. (1988) 'Denial and confirmatory search; paradoxical consequences of medical diagnosis', *Journal of Applied Social Psychology* 18, 473–90.

Da Costa, J. M. (1871) 'On irritable heart: a clinical study of a form of functional cardiac disorder and its consequences', *American Journal of Medical Science* 121, 2052.

Dainty, E. (1988) 'M.E. and I', *Nursing Standard* 84, 49–50.

David, A., Pelosi, A., McDonald, E., Stephens, D., Ledger, D., Rathbone, R. and Mann, A. (1990) 'Tired, weak, or in need of rest: fatigue among general practice attenders', *British Medical Journal* 301, 1199–202.

David, A. and Wessely, S. (1993) 'Chronic fatigue, ME, and ICD-10', *Lancet* 342, 1247–8.

Davison, K. P. and Pennebaker, J. W. (1997) 'Virtual narratives: illness representations in online support groups', in K. J. Petrie and J. Weinman (eds) *Perceptions of Health and Illness*, London: Harwood Academic.

De Lorenzo, F., Xiao, H., Mukherjee, M., Harcup, J., Suleiman, S., Kadziola, Z. and Kakkar, V. V. (1998) 'Chronic fatigue syndrome: physical and cardiovascular deconditioning', *Quarterly Journal of Medicine* 91(7), 475–81.

Deale, A., Chalder, T., Marks, I. and Wessely, S. (1997) 'Cognitive behavior therapy for chronic fatigue syndrome: a randomized controlled trial', *American Journal of Psychiatry* 154(3), 408–14.

Deale, A., Chalder, T. and Wessely, S. (1998) 'Illness beliefs and treatment outcome in chronic fatigue syndrome', *Journal of Psychosomatic Research* 45(1 Spec No), 77–83.

Deirdre (1990) Meeting members page, *Meeting-Place* 34, 32.

Demitrack, M. A. (1993) 'Chronic fatigue syndrome: A disease of the hypo-thalamic–pituitary–adrenal axis?', *Annals of Medicine* 26, 1–5.

Demitrack, M. A. (1996) 'The psychobiology of chronic fatigue: the central nervous system as a final common pathway', in M. A. Demitrack and S. E. Abbey (eds), *Chronic Fatigue Syndrome: An Integrated Approach to Evaluation and Treatment*, New York: Guilford Press.

Demitrack, M. A. and Abbey, S. E. (1996) 'Historical overview and evolu-tion of contemporary definitions of chronic fatigue states', in M. A. Demitrack and S. E. Abbey (eds), *Chronic Fatigue Syndrome: An Inte-grated Approach to Evaluation and Treatment*, New York: Guilford Press.

Demitrack, M. A., Dale, J. K., Straus, S. E., Laue, L., Listwak, S. J., Kruesi, M. J., Chrousos, G. P. and Gold, P. W. (1991) 'Evidence for impaired acti-vation of the hypothalamic–pituitary–adrenal axis in patients with chronic fatigue syndrome', *Journal of Clinical Endocrinology and Metabolism* 73(6), 1224–34.

Dinan, T. G., Majeed, T., Lavelle, E., Scott, L. V., Berti, C. and Behan, P. (1997) 'Blunted serotonin-mediated activation of the hypothalamic–pituitary–adrenal axis in chronic fatigue syndrome', *Psychoneuroendo-crinology* 22(4), 261–7.

Djaldetti, R., Ziv, I., Achiron, A. and Melamed, E. (1996) 'Fatigue in multiple sclerosis compared with chronic fatigue syndrome: a quantitative assessment', *Neurology* 46(3), 632–5.

Dopperpuhl, H. (1998) 'One day at a time', *Meeting-Place* 55, 37.

Dowsett, E. (1990) quoted in S. Stacey 'Tired and tested', October *Harpers and Queen*.

Dunnell, K. and Cartwright, A. (1972) *Medicine takers, prescribers and hoarders*, London: Routledge.

Dwyer, J. M. (1988) *The Body at War*, Sydney: Allen & Unwin.

Edwards, R. H., Gibson, H., Clague, J. E. and Helliwell, T. (1993) 'Muscle histopathology and physiology in chronic fatigue syndrome', *Ciba Foun-dation Symposium* 173, 102–17; discussion 117–31.

Euga, R., Chalder, T., Deale, A. and Wessely, S. (1996) 'A comparison of the characteristics of chronic fatigue syndrome in primary and tertiary care', *British Journal of Psychiatry* 168(1), 121–6.

Farmer, A., Jones, I., Hillier, J., Llewelyn, M., Borysiewicz, L.K. and Smith, A. (1995) 'Neurasthenia revisited: ICD-10 and DSM-III-R psychiatric syndromes in chronic fatigue patients and comparison subjects', *British Journal of Psychiatry* 167, 503–6.

Fiedler, N., Kipen, H. M., DeLuca, J., Kelly-McNeil, K. and Natelson, B. (1996) 'A controlled comparison of multiple chemical sensitivities and chronic fatigue syndrome', *Psychosomatic Medicine* 58, 38–49.

Fielding, R. A., Manfredi, T. J., Ding, W., Fiatarone, M. A., Evans, W. J. and Cannon, J. G. (1993) 'Acute phase response in exercise: III. Neutrophil and IL-1 beta accumulation in skeletal muscle', *American Journal of Physiology* 265, 166–72.

Fischler, B., Cluydts, R., De Gucht, Y., Kaufman, L. and De Meirleir, K. (1997a) 'Generalized anxiety disorder in chronic fatigue syndrome', *Acta Psychiatrica Scandinavica* 95(5), 405–13.

Fischler, B., Dendale, P., Michiels, V., Cluydts, R., Kaufman, L. and De Meirleir, K. (1997b) 'Physical fatigability and exercise capacity in chronic fatigue syndrome: association with disability, somatization and psychopathology', *Journal of Psychosomatic Research* 42(4), 369–78.

Fischler, B., D'Haenen, H., Cluydts, R., Michiels, V., Demets, K., Bossuyt, A., Kaufman, L. and De Meirleir, K. (1996) 'Comparison of 99m Tc HMPAO SPECT scan between chronic fatigue syndrome, major depression and healthy controls: an exploratory study of clinical correlates of regional cerebral blood flow', *Neuropsychobiology* 34(4), 175–83.

Fischler, B., Le Bon, O., Hoffmann, G., Cluydts, R., Kaufman, L. and De Meirleir, K. (1997c) 'Sleep anomalies in the chronic fatigue syndrome. A comorbidity study', *Neuropsychobiology* 35(3), 115–22.

Fone, D. L., Constantine, C. E. and McCloskey, B. (1998) 'The Worcester water incident, UK: bias in self reported symptoms to an emergency helpline', *Journal of Epidemiology and Community Health* 52, 526–7.

Frazer, D. (1995) 'Living with CFS/ME', *Meeting-Place* 45, 17–18.

Freeman, R. and Komaroff, A. L. (1997) 'Does the chronic fatigue syndrome involve the autonomic nervous system?', *American Journal of Medicine*, 102, 357–64.

Freese, C. H. (1991) Letter from the editor, *CFIDS Chronicle*, 1, ii.

Friedberg, F. and Krupp, L. B. (1994) 'A comparison of cognitive behavioral treatment for chronic fatigue syndrome and primary depression', *Clinical Infectious Diseases* 18(Suppl. 1), S105–10.

Frost, K., Frank, E. and Maibach, E. (1997) 'Relative risk in the news media: a quantification of misrepresentation', *American Journal of Public Health* 87, 842–5.

Fry, A. M. and Martin, M. A. (1996a) 'Cognitive idiosyncrasies among children with the chronic fatigue syndrome: anomalies in self-reported activity levels', *Journal of Psychosomatic Research* 41, 213–23.

Fry, A. M. and Martin, M. A. (1996b) 'Fatigue in the chronic fatigue syndrome: a cognitive phenomenon?', *Journal of Psychosomatic Research* 41, 415–26.

Fukuda, K., Straus, S. E., Hickie, I., Sharpe, M. C., Dobbins, J. G. and Komaroff, A. (1994) 'The chronic fatigue syndrome: a comprehensive approach to its definition and study', International Chronic Fatigue Syndrome Study Group, *Annals of Internal Medicine* 121(12), 953–9.

Fulcher, K. Y. and White, P. D. (1997) 'Randomised controlled trial of graded exercise in patients with the chronic fatigue syndrome', *British Medical Journal* 314(7095), 1647–52.

Goldenberg, D. L., Simms, R. W., Geiger, A. and Komaroff, A. L. (1990) 'High frequency of fibromyalgia in patients with chronic fatigue seen in a primary care practice', *Arthritis and Rheumatism* 33, 381–7.

Goldstein, J. A. (1993) *Betrayal by the brain*, New York: Harwood Medical Press.

Goldstein, J., Mena, I., Jouanne, E. and Lesser, I. (1995) 'The assessment of vascular abnormalities in late life chronic fatigue syndrome by brain SPECT: comparison with late life major depressive disorder', *Journal of Chronic Fatigue Syndrome* 1, 55–79.

Gonder-Frederick, L. and Cox, D. J. (1991) 'Symptom perception, symptom beliefs, and blood glucose discrimination in the self treatment of insulin dependent diabetes', in J. A. Skelton and R. T. Croyle (eds), *Mental Representations in Health and Illness*, New York: Springer-Verlag.

Grafman, J., Schwartz, V., Dale, J. K., Scheffers, M., Houser, C. and Straus, S. E. (1993) 'Analysis of neuropsychological functioning in patients with chronic fatigue syndrome', *Journal of Neurology, Neurosurgery and Psychiatry* 56(6), 684–9.

Gray, G. C., Kaiser, K. S., Hawksworth, A. W., Hall, F. W. and Barrett-Connor, E. (1999) 'Increased postwar symptoms and psychological morbidity among US Navy Gulf War veterans', *American Journal of Tropical Medicine and Hygiene* 60(5), 758–66.

Greenberg, D. B. (1990) 'Neurasthenia in the 1980s: chronic mononucleosis, chronic fatigue syndrome, and anxiety and depressive disorders', *Psychosomatics* 31(2), 129–37.

Greg (1991–1992) 'Dear Meeting-Place', *Meeting-Place* 37, 35.

Gruber, A. J., Hudson, J. I. and Pope, H. G. (1996) 'The management of treatment-resistant depression in disorders on the interface of psychiatry and medicine', *Psychiatric Clinics of North America* 19, 351–69.

Gunn, W. J., Connell, D. B. and Randall, B. (1993) 'Epidemiology of chronic fatigue syndrome: The Centre for Disease Control study', *Ciba Foundation Symposium* 173, 83–101.

Gupta, S. and Vayuvegula, B. (1991) 'A comprehensive immunological analysis in chronic fatigue syndrome', *Scandinavian Journal of Immunology* 33, 319–27.

Hannay, D. R. (1978) 'Symptom prevalence in the community', *Journal of the Royal College of General Practitioners* 28, 492–9.

Hassan, I. S., Bannister, B. A., Akbar, A., Weor, W. and Bofill, M. (1998) 'A study of the immunology of the chronic fatigue syndrome – correlation of immunological parameters to health dysfunction', *Clinical Immunology and Immunopathology* 87, 60–7.

Haynes, R. B., Sackett, D. L., Taylor, W., Gibson, E. S. and Johnson, A. L. (1978) 'Increased absenteeism from work after detection and labeling of hypertensive patients', *New England Journal of Medicine* 299, 741–4.

Heijmans, M. J. (1998) 'Coping and adaptive outcome in chronic fatigue syndrome: importance of illness cognitions', *Journal of Psychosomatic Research* 45, 39–51.

Heijmans, M., de Ridder, D. and Bensing, J. (1999) 'Dissimilarity in patients' and spouses' representations of chronic illness: exploration of relations to patient adaptation', *Psychology and Health* 14, 451–66.

Heijmans, M. and de Ridder, D. (1998) 'Assessing illness representations of chronic illness: explorations of their disease-specific nature', *Journal of Behavioral Medicine* 21, 485–503.

Hellinger, W. C., Smith, T. F., Van Scoy, R. E., Spitzer, P. G., Forgas, P. and Edson, R. S. (1988) 'Chronic fatigue syndrome and the diagnostic utility of antibody to Epstein–Barr virus early antigen', *Journal of the American Medical Association* 260, 971–3.

Henderson, D. A. and Shelkov, A. (1959) 'Epidemic neuromyasthenia – clinical syndrome?', *New England Journal of Medicine* 260, 757–64, 814–8.

Henle, G., Henle, W. and Diehl, V. (1968) 'Relation of Burkitt's tumorassociated herpes-type virus to infectious mononucleosis', *Proceedings of the National Academy of Sciences of the United States of America* 59(1), 94–101.

Hickie, I., Bennet, A., Lloyd, A., Heath, A. and Martin, N. (1999) 'Complex genetic and enviromental relationships between psychological distress, fatigue and immune functioning: a twin study', *Psychological Medicine* 29(5), 269–77.

Hickie, I., Lloyd, A., Hadzi-Pavlovic, D., Parker, G., Bird, K. and Wakefield, D. (1995) 'Can the chronic fatigue syndrome be defined by distinct clinical features?', *Psychological Medicine* 25(5), 925–35.

Hickie, I., Lloyd, A., Wakefield, D. and Parker, G. (1990) 'The psychiatric status of patients with the chronic fatigue syndrome', *British Journal of Psychiatry* 156, 534–40.

Holmes, G. P., Kaplan, J. E., Gantz, N. M., Komaroff, A. L., Schonberger, L. B., Straus, S. E., Jones, J. F., Dubois, R. E., Cunningham-Rundles, C., Pahwa, S., Tosato, G., Zegans, L. S., Purtilo, D. T., Brown, N., Schooley, R. T. and Brus, I. (1988) 'Chronic fatigue syndrome: a working case definition', *Annals of Internal Medicine* 108(3), 387–9.

Holmes, G. P., Kaplan, J. E., Stewart, J. A., Hunt, B., Pinsky, P. F. and Schonberger, L. B. (1987) 'A cluster of patients with a chronic mononucleosis-like syndrome. Is Epstein–Barr virus the cause?', *Journal of the American Medical Association* 257(17), 2297–302.

Hopwood, D. G. and Guidotti, T. L. (1988) 'Recall bias in exposed subjects following a toxic exposure incident', *Archives of Environmental Health* 43, 234–7.

Horne, S. (1992) *M.E.rely triumphant,* unpublished Master's thesis, Massey University, Palmerston North.

Hotchin, N. A., Read, R., Smith, D. G. and Crawford, D. H. (1989) 'Active Epstein–Barr virus infection in postviral fatigue syndrome', *Journal of Infection* 18, 143–50.

Hotopf, M., Noah, N. and Wessely, S. (1996) 'Chronic fatigue and minor psychiatric morbidity after viral meningitis: a controlled study', *Journal of Neurology, Neurosurgery and Psychiatry* 60(5), 504–9.

Ho-Yen, D. and McNamara, I. (1991) 'General practitioners' experience of chronic fatigue syndrome', *British Journal of General Practice* 41, 324–6.

Hudson, J. I. and Pope, H. G. (1994) 'The concept of affective spectrum disorder: relationship to fibromyalgia and other syndromes of chronic fatigue and chronic muscle pain', *Baillière's Clinical Rheumatology* 8, 839–56.

Hyams, K. C. (1998a) 'Lessons derived from evaluating Gulf War Syndrome – suggested guidelines for investigating possible outbreaks of new diseases', *Psychosomatic Medicine* 60(2), 137–9.

Hyams, K. C. (1998b) 'Developing case definitions for symptom-based conditions: the problem of specificity', *Epidemiological Reviews* 20, 148–56.

Hyams, K. C., Wignall, S. and Roswell, R. (1996) 'War syndromes and their evaluation: from the US Civil War to the Persian Gulf War', *Annals of Internal Medicine* 125, 396–405.

Imboden, J. B., Canter, A. and Cluff, L. E. (1961) 'Convalescence from influenza: a study of the psychological and clinical determinants', *Archives of Internal Medicine* 108, 115–21.

Imboden, J. B., Canter, A., Cluff, L. E. and Trever, R. W. (1959) 'Brucellosis III. Psychological aspects of delayed convalescence', *Archives of Internal Medicine* 103, 78–86.

Ingram, R. E. (1990) 'Self-focused attention in clinical disorders: review and a conceptual model', *Psychological Bulletin* 107, 156–76.

Irwin, M., Mascovich, A., Gillin, J. C., Willoughby, R., Pike, J. and Smith, T. L. (1994) 'Partial sleep deprivation reduces natural killer cell activity in humans', *Psychosomatic Medicine* 56, 493–8.

Isaacs, R. (1948) 'Chronic infectious mononucleosis', *Blood* 3, 858–61.

Ismail, K., Everitt, B., Blatchley, N., Hull, L., Unwin, C., David, A. and Wessely, S. (1999) 'Is there a Gulf War syndrome?', *Lancet* 353(9148), 179–82.

Jauchem, J. R. (1992) 'Epidemiological studies of electric and magnetic fields and cancer: a case study of distortions by the media', *Journal of Clinical Epidemiology* 45, 1137–42.

Jefferies, W. (1994) 'Mild adrenocortical deficiency, chronic allergies, auto-immune disorders and the chronic fatigue syndrome: a continuation of the cortisone story', *Medical Hypotheses* 42, 183–9.

Jemmott, J. B. D., Ditto, P. H. and Croyle, R. T. (1986) 'Judging health status: effects of perceived prevalence and personal relevance', *Journal of Personality and Social Psycholology* 50(5), 899–905.

Johnson, S. K., Deluca, J. and Natelson, B. H. (1996a) 'Depression in fatiguing illness – comparing patients with chronic fatigue syndrome, multiple sclerosis and depression', *Journal of Affective Disorders* 39(1), 21–30.

Johnson, S. K., Deluca, J. and Natelson, B. H. (1996b) 'Assessing somatization disorder in the chronic fatigue syndrome', *Psychosomatic Medicine* 58(1), 50–7.

Johnson, S. K., Deluca, J. and Natelson, B. H. (1996c) 'Personality dimensions in the chronic fatigue syndrome: a comparison with multiple sclerosis and depression', *Journal of Psychiatric Research* 30, 9–20.

Jones, J. F., Ray, C. G., Minnich, L. L., Hicks, M. J., Kibler, R. and Lucas, D. O. (1985) 'Evidence for active Epstein–Barr virus infection in patients with persistent, unexplained illnesses: elevated anti-early antigen antibodies', *Annals of Internal Medicine* 102(1), 1–7.

Joyce, E., Blumenthal, S. and Wessely, S. (1996) 'Memory, attention, and executive function in chronic fatigue syndrome', *Journal of Neurology, Neurosurgery and Psychiatry* 60(5), 495–503.

Joyce, J., Hotopf, M. and Wessely, S. (1997) 'The prognosis of chronic fatigue and chronic fatigue syndrome: a systematic review', *Quarterly Journal of Medicine* 90(3), 223–33.

Judy (1991) 'The Nine-Year Nightmare', *Meeting-Place* 35, 38–42.

Kasl, S. V., Evans, A. S. and Niederman, J. C. (1979) 'Psychosocial risk factors in the development of infectious mononucleosis', *Psychosomatic Medicine* 41(6), 445–66.

Katon, W. and Russo, J. (1992) 'Chronic fatigue symptom criteria. A critique of the requirement for multiple physical complaints', *Archives of Internal Medicine* 152, 1604–16.

Katon, W. J., Buchwald, D. S., Simon, G. E., Russo, J. E. and Mease, P. J. (1991) 'Psychiatric illness in patients with chronic fatigue and those with rheumatoid arthritis', *Journal of General Internal Medicine* 6, 277–85.

Kawai, K. and Kawai, A. (1992) 'Studies on the relationship between chronic fatigue syndrome and Epstein–Barr virus in Japan', *Internal Medicine* 31, 313–8.

Keefe, F. J., Brown, G. K., Wallston, K. A. and Caldwell, D. S. (1989) 'Coping with rheumatoid arthritis pain: catastrophizing as a maladaptive strategy', *Pain* 37, 51–6.

Kirmayer, L. J. and Robbins, J. M. (1991) 'Functional somatic symptoms', in L. J. Kirmayer and J. M. Robbins (eds), *Current Concepts of Somatization:*

Research and Clinical Perspectives, Washington: American Psychiatric Press.

Kleinman, A. I. (1993) 'In conclusion', *Ciba Foundation Symposium* 173, 342–5.

Klimas, N. G., Salvato, F. R., Morgan, R. and Fletcher, M. A. (1990) 'Immunologic abnormalities in chronic fatigue syndrome', *Journal of Clinical Microbiology* 28(6), 1403–10.

Komaroff, A. L. and Buchwald, D. (1991) 'Symptoms and signs of chronic fatigue syndrome', *Reviews of Infectious Diseases* 13(Suppl. 1), S8–11.

Komaroff, A. L., Fagioli, L. R., Doolittle, T. H., Gandek, B., Gleit, M. A., Guerriero, R. T., Kornish, R. J., II, Ware, N. C., Ware, J. E., Jr. and Bates, D. W. (1996) 'Health status in patients with chronic fatigue syndrome and in general population and disease comparison groups', *American Journal of Medicine* 101(3), 281–90.

Kroenke, K. (1998) 'Gender differences in the reporting of physical and somatoform symptoms', *Psychosomatic Medicine* 60, 150–55.

Kronfol, Z., House, J. D., Silva, J. J., Greden, J. and Carroll, B. J. (1986) 'Depression, urinary free cortisol excretion and lymphocyte function', *British Journal of Psychiatry* 148, 70–3.

Krupp, L. B. and Pollina, D. (1996) 'Neuroimmune and neuropsychiatric aspects of chronic fatigue syndrome', *Advances in Neuroimmunology* 6, 155–67.

Landay, A. L., Jessop, C., Lennette, E. T. and Levy, J. A. (1991) 'Chronic fatigue syndrome: clinical condition associated with immune activation', *Lancet* 338, 701–12.

Lane, T. J., Manu, P. and Matthews, D. (1991) 'Depression and somatization in the chronic fatigue syndrome', *American Journal of Medicine* 91, 335–43.

Lavietes, M. H., Natelson, B. H., Cordero, D. L., Ellis, S. P. and Tapp, W. N. (1996) 'Does the stressed patient with chronic fatigue syndrome hyperventilate?', *International Journal of Behavioral Medicine* 3(1), 70–83.

Lawrie, S. M., MacHale, S. M., Power, M. J. and Goodwin, G. M. (1997) 'Chronic fatigue syndrome and sense of effort', *Psychological Medicine* 27, 995–9.

Lawrie, S. M. and Pelosi, A. J. (1995) 'Chronic fatigue syndrome in the community: prevalence and associations', *British Journal of Psychiatry* 166, 793–7.

Lee, S. (1994) 'Neurasthenia and Chinese psychiatry in the 1990s', *Journal of Psychosomatic Research* 38, 487–91.

Leese, G., Chattington, P., Fraser, W., Vora, J., Edwards, R. and Williams, G. (1996) 'Short-term night-shift working mimics the pituitary-adrenocortical dysfunction in chronic fatigue syndrome', *Journal of Clinical Endocrinology and Metabolism* 81(5), 1867–70.

Leventhal, H., Meyer, D. and Nerenz, D. (1980) 'The common sense representation of illness danger', in S. Rachman (ed), *Contributions to Medical*

Psychology, New York: Pergamon Press.

Leventhal, H., Nerenz, D. R. and Steele, D. J. (1984) 'Illness representations and coping with health threats', in A. Baum and J. Singer (eds), *A Handbook of Psychology and Health* Vol. 4, Hillsdale: NJ: Erlbaum.

Levine, P. H. (1997) 'Epidemiologic advances in chronic fatigue syndrome', *Journal of Psychiatric Research* 31(1), 7–18.

Levy, J. A. (1994) 'Viral studies of chronic fatigue syndrome', *Clinical Infectious Diseases* 18(Suppl. 1), S117– 20.

Lewis, G. and Wessely, S. (1992) 'The epidemiology of fatigue: more questions than answers', *Journal of Epidemiology and Community Health* 46(2), 92–7.

Lewis, S., Cooper, C. L. and Bennett, D. (1994) 'Psychosocial factors and chronic fatigue syndrome', *Psychological Medicine* 24, 661–71.

Lloyd, A., Hickie, I., Hickie, C., Dwyer, J. and Wakefield, D. (1992) 'Cell-mediated immunity in patients with chronic fatigue syndrome, healthy control subjects and patients with major depression', *Clinical and Experimental Immunology* 87(1), 76–9.

Lloyd, A. R., Gandevia, S., Brockman, A., Hales, J. and Wakefield, D. (1994) 'Cytokine production and fatigue in patients with chronic fatigue syndrome and healthy control subjects in response to exercise', *Clinical Infectious Diseases* 18(Suppl. 1), S142–6.

Lloyd, A. R., Hickie, I., Boughton, C. R., Spencer, O. and Wakefield, D. (1990) 'Prevalence of chronic fatigue syndrome in an Australian population', *Medical Journal of Australia* 153(9), 522–8.

Lloyd, A. R., Hickie, I., Brockman, A., Hickie, C., Wilson, A., Dwyer, J. and Wakefield, D. (1993) 'Immunologic and psychologic therapy for patients with chronic fatigue syndrome: a double-blind, placebo-controlled trial', *American Journal of Medicine* 94(2), 197–203.

Lloyd, A. R., Hickie, I. and Gandevia, S. C. (1988a) 'Muscle strength, endurance and recovery in the post-infection fatigue syndrome', *Journal of Neurology, Neurosurgery and Psychiatry* 51, 1316–22.

Lloyd, A. R. and Pender, H. (1992) 'The economic impact of chronic fatigue syndrome', *Medical Journal of Australia* 157, 599–601.

Lloyd, A. R., Wakefield, D., Boughton, C. R. and Dwyer, J. (1988b) 'What is myalgic encephalomyelitis?', *Lancet* 1, 1286–7.

Lopez, J. (1991) 'What's eating you', *Meeting-Place* 35, 12–13.

Lopis, R. (1995) 'Living with CFS/ME', *Meeting-Place* 45, 15–17.

Lutgendorf, S. K., Antoni, M., Ironson, G., Fletcher, M., Penedo, F., Baum, A., Schneiderman, N. and Klimas, N. (1995) 'Physical symptoms of chronic fatigue are exacerbated by the stress of Hurricane Andrew', *Psychosomatic Medicine* 57, 310–23.

McCully, K. K., Natelson, B. H., Iotti, S., Sisto, S. and Leigh, J. S., Jr. (1996a) 'Reduced oxidative muscle metabolism in chronic fatigue syndrome', *Muscle and Nerve* 19(5), 621–5.

McCully, K. K., Sisto, S. A. and Natelson, B. H. (1996b) 'Use of exercise for treatment of chronic fatigue syndrome', *Sports Medicine* 21(1), 35–48.

McDonald, E., Cope, H. and David, A. (1993a) 'Cognitive impairment in patients with chronic fatigue: a preliminary study', *Journal of Neurology, Neurosurgery and Psychiatry* 56(7), 812–5.

McDonald, E., David, A. S., Pelosi, A. J. and Mann, A. (1993b) 'Chronic fatigue in primary care attenders', *Psychological Medicine* 23, 987–98.

MacDonald, K. L., Osterholm, M. T., LeDell, K., White, K., Schenck, C. H. and Chao, C. C. (1996) 'A case–controlled study to assess possible triggers and cofactors in chronic fatigue syndrome', *American Journal of Medicine* 100, 548–54.

McEvedy, C. P. and Beard, A. W. (1970a) 'Royal Free epidemic of 1955: a reconstruction', *British Medical Journal* 1, 7–11.

McEvedy, C. P. and Beard, A. W. (1970b) 'Concept of benign myalgic encephalomyelitis', *British Medical Journal* 1, 11–15.

Macfarlane, J. G., Shahal, B., Mously, C. and Moldofsky, H. (1996) 'Periodic K-alpha sleep EEG activity and periodic limb movements during sleep – comparisons of clinical features and sleep parameters', *Sleep* 19(3), 200–4.

McGregor, N. R., Dunstan, R. H., Zerbes, M., Butt, H. L., Roberts, T. K. and Klineberg, I. J. (1996a) 'Preliminary determination of a molecular basis of chronic fatigue syndrome', *Biochemical and Molecular Medicine* 57(2), 73–80.

McGregor, N. R., Dunstan, R. H., Zerbes, M., Butt, H. L., Roberts, T. K. and Klineberg, I. J. (1996b) 'Preliminary determination of the association between symptom expression and urinary metabolites in subjects with chronic fatigue syndrome', *Biochemical and Molecular Medicine* 58(1), 85–92.

MacHale, S. M., Cavanagh, J. T., Bennie, J., Carroll, S., Goodwin, G. M. and Lawrie, S. M. (1998) 'Diurnal variation of adrenocortical activity in chronic fatigue syndrome', *Neuropsychobiology* 38(4), 213–7.

McKenzie, R., O'Fallon, A., Dale, J., Demitrack, M., Sharma, G., Deloria, M., Garcia-Borreguero, D., Blackwelder, W. and Straus, S. E. (1998) 'Low-dose hydrocortisone for treatment of chronic fatigue syndrome: a randomized controlled trial', *Journal of the American Medical Association* 280(12), 1061–6.

MacLean, G. and Wessely, S. (1994) 'Professional and popular views of chronic fatigue syndrome', *British Medical Journal* 308(6931), 776–7.

McMahan, S. and Meyer, J. (1995) 'Symptom prevalence and worry about high voltage transmission lines', *Environmnetal Research* 70, 114–8.

Magnusson, A. E., Nias, D. K. and White, P. D. (1996) 'Is perfectionism associated with fatigue?', *Journal of Psychosomatic Research* 41(4), 377–83.

Manu, P., Lane, T. J. and Mathews, D. A. (1988) 'The frequency of the chronic fatigue syndrome in patients with symptoms of persistent fatigue', *Annals of Internal Medicine* 109, 554–6.

Manu, P., Lane, T. J. and Mathews, D. A. (1993a) 'Chronic fatigue and chronic fatigue syndrome: clinical epidemiology and aetiological classification', in E. Bock and J. Whelan (eds) *Chronic fatigue syndrome*, Ciba Foundation Symposium (Vol. 173).

Manu, P., Lane, T. J., Matthews, D. A., Castriotta, R. J., Watson, R. K. and Abeles, M. (1994) 'Alpha-delta sleep in patients with a chief complaint of chronic fatigue', *Southern Medical Journal* 87(4), 465–70.

Manu, P., Matthews, D. A. and Lane, T. J. (1993b) 'Food intolerance in patients with chronic fatigue', *International Journal of Eating Disorders* 13(2), 203–9.

Marshal, P. S., Forstot, M., Callies, A., Peterson, P. K. and Schenck, C. H. (1997) 'Cognitive slowing and working memory difficulties in chronic fatigue syndrome', *Psychosomatic Medicine* 59, 58–66.

Masuda, A., Nozoe, S. I., Matsuyama, T. and Tanaka, H. (1994) 'Psychobehavioural and immunological characteristics of adult people with chronic fatigue and patients with chronic fatigue syndrome', *Psychosomatic Medicine* 56, 512–8.

Mathews, D. A., Lane, T. J. and Manu, P. (1991) 'Antibodies to Epstein–Barr virus in patients with chronic fatigue', *South African Medical Journal* 84, 832–40.

Mawle, A. C., Nisenbaum, R., Dobbins, J. G., Gary, H. E., Stewart, J. A., Reyes, M., L., S., Schmid, D. S. and Reeves, W. C. (1997) 'Immune responses associated with chronic fatigue syndrome – a case–control study', *Journal of Infectious Diseases* 175, 136–41.

Meeting-Place (1990) 'A tale of three press releases … ', *Meeting-Place* 31, 30–31.

Meeting-Place (1996) 'CFIDS Association Conference', *Meeting-Place* 46, 23.

Millon, C., Salvato, F., Blaney, N., Morgan, R., Mantero-Atienza, E., Klimas, N. and Fletcher, M. (1989) 'A psychological assessment of chronic fatigue syndrome/chronic Epstein–Barr virus patients', *Psychology and Health* 31, 31–41.

Morris, D. H. and Stare, F. J. (1993) 'Unproven diet therapies in the treatment of the chronic fatigue syndrome', *Archives of Family Medicine* 2(2), 181–6.

Morriss, R., Sharpe, M., Sharpley, A. L., Cowen, P. J., Hawton, K. and Morris, J. (1993) 'Abnormalities of sleep in patients with the chronic fatigue syndrome', *British Medical Journal* 306(6886), 1161–4.

Moss-Morris, R. (1997) *Cognitive factors in the maintenance of chronic fatigue syndrome.* Unpublished PhD, University of Auckland, Auckland.

Moss-Morris, R. (1997a) 'Epstein–Barr virus infection', in A. Baum, C. McManus, S. Newman, J. Weinman and R. West (eds), *Cambridge Handbook of Psychology, Health and Medicine*, Cambridge: Cambridge University Press.

Moss-Morris, R. (1997b) 'The role of illness cognitions and coping in the aetiology and maintenance of the chronic fatigue syndrome', in K. J. Petrie and J. Weinman (eds) *Perceptions of Health and Illness*, London: Harwood Academic.

Moss-Morris, R. and Petrie, K. J. (1997) 'Cognitive distortions of somatic experiences – revision and validation of a measure', *Journal of Psychosomatic Research* 43(3), 293–306.

Moss-Morris, R. and Petrie, K. J. (1999) 'Link between psychiatric dysfunction and dizziness', *Lancet* 353, 515–6.

Moss-Morris, R., Petrie, K. J., Large, R. G. and Kydd, R. R. (1996a) 'Neuropsychological deficits in chronic fatigue syndrome – artifact or reality', *Journal of Neurology, Neurosurgery and Psychiatry* 60(5), 474–7.

Moss-Morris, R., Petrie, K. J. and Weinman, J. (1996b) 'Functioning in chronic fatigue syndrome – do illness perceptions play a regulatory role?', *British Journal of Health Psychology 1* (Part 1), 15–25.

Murdoch, J. C. (1988) 'The myalgic encephalomyelitis syndrome', *Family Practice* 5, 302–6.

Murphy, H., Dickens, C., Creed, F. and Bernstein, R. (1999) 'Depression, illness perception and coping in rheumatoid arthritis', *Journal of Psychosomatic Research* 46, 155–164.

Natelson, B. H., Cheu, J., Pareja, J., Ellis, S. P., Policastro, T. and Findley, T. W. (1996) 'Randomized, double blind, controlled placebo-phase in trial of low dose phenelzine in the chronic fatigue syndrome', *Psychopharmacology* 124(3), 226–30.

Natelson, B. H., Cohen, J. M., Brassloff, I. and Lee, H. J. (1993) 'A controlled study of brain magnetic resonance imaging in patients with the chronic fatigue syndrome', *Journal of the Neurological Sciences* 120(2), 213–7.

Natelson, B. H., Ellis, S. P., Braonain, P. J., DeLuca, J. and Tapp, W. N. (1995) 'Frequency of deviant immunological test values in chronic fatigue syndrome patients', *Clinical and Diagnostic Laboratory Immunology* 2(2), 238–40.

Nerenz, D. R., Leventhal, H. and Love, R. R. (1982) 'Factors contributing to emotional distress during cancer chemotherapy', *Cancer* 50(5), 1020–7.

Parker, S. L., Garner, D. M., Leznoff, A., Sussman, G. L. *et al.* (1991) 'Psychological characteristics of patients with reported adverse reactions to food', *International Journal of Eating Disorders* 10(4), 433–9.

Pawlikowska, T., Chalder, T., Hirsch, S. R., Wallace, P., Wright, D. J. M. and Wessely, S. C. (1994) 'Population based study of fatigue and psychological distress', *British Medical Journal* 308, 763–308.

Peakman, M., Deale, A., Field, R., Mahalingam, M. and Wessely, S. (1997)

'Clinical improvement in chronic fatigue syndrome is not associated with lymphocyte subsets of function or activation', *Clinical Immunology and Immunopathology* 82(1), 83–91.

Pennebaker, J. W. (1982) *The Psychology of Physical Symptoms*, New York: Springer-Verlag.

Pepper, C., Krupp, L., Friedberg, F., Doscher, C. and Coyle, P. (1993) 'A comparison of neuropsychiatric characteristics in chronic fatigue syndrome, multiple sclerosis and major depression', *Journal of Neuropsychiatry Clinical Neurosciences* 5, 200–5.

Peterson, P. K., Sirr, S. A., Grammith, F. C., Schenck, C. H., Pheley, A. M., Hu, S. and Chao, C. C. (1994) 'Effects of mild exercise on cytokines and cerebral blood flow in chronic fatigue syndrome patients', *Clinical and Diagnostic Laboratory Immunology* 1, 222–6.

Petrie, K. J., Booth, R. J., Elder, H. and Cameron, L. D. (1999) 'Psychological influences on the perception of imune function', *Psychological Medicine* 29, 391–7.

Petrie, K. J. and Moss-Morris, R. (1997) 'Coping with chronic illness', in A. Baum, S. Newman, J. Weinman, R. West and C. McManus (eds), *Cambridge Handbook of Psychology, Health and Medicine*, Cambridge: Cambridge University Press.

Petrie, K. J., Moss-Morris, R. and Weinman, J. (1995) 'Catastrophic beliefs and their implications in the chronic fatigue syndrome', *Journal of Psychosomatic Research* 39, 31–7.

Petrie, K. J. and Weinman, J. (1997a) 'Illness representations and recovery from myocardial infarction', in K. J. Petrie and J. Weinman (eds), *Perceptions of Health and Illness*, London: Harwood Academic.

Petrie, K. J., Weinman, J., Sharpe, N. and Buckley, J. (1996) 'Role of patients' view of their illness in predicting return to work and functioning after myocardial infarction – longitudinal study', *British Medical Journal* 312(7040), 1191–4.

Petrie, K. J. and Weinman, J. A. (eds) (1997b) *Perceptions of Health and Illness*, London: Harwood Academic.

Poore, M., Snow, P. and Paul, C. (1984) 'An unexplained illness in West Otago. *New Zealand Medical Journal* 97, 351–4.

Price, R. K., North, C. S., Wessely, S. and Fraser, V. J. (1992) 'Estimating the prevalence of chronic fatigue syndrome and associated symptoms in the community', *Public Health Reports* 107(5), 514–22.

Pruessner, J. C., Helhammer, D. H. and Kirschbaum, C. (1999) 'Burnout, perceived stress, and cortisol responses to awakening', *Psychosomatic Medicine* 61, 197–204.

Ray, C. (1991) 'Chronic fatigue syndrome and depression: conceptual and methodological ambiguities' (editorial), *Psychological Medicine* 21(1), 1–9.

Ray, C., Jefferies, S. and Weir, W. R. (1997) 'Coping and other predictors of outcome in chronic fatigue syndrome: a 1-year follow-up', *Journal of Psychosomatic Research* 43(4), 405–15.

Ray, C., Jefferies, S., Weir, W. R., Hayes, K., Simon, S. F. A. and Marriot, P. (1998) 'Making sense of chronic fatigue syndrome: patients' accounts of onset', *Psychology and Health* 13, 99–109.

Ray, C., Jefferies, S. and Weir, W. R. C. (1995) 'Coping with chronic fatigue syndrome: illness responses and their relationship with fatigue, functional impairment and emotional status', *Psychological Medicine* 25(5), 937–45.

Ray, C., Phillips, L. and Weir, W. R. (1993a) 'Quality of attention in chronic fatigue syndrome: subjective reports of everyday attention and cognitive difficulty, and performance on tasks of focused attention', *British Journal of Clinical Psychology* 32(Pt 3), 357–64.

Ray, C., Weir, W., Stewart, D., Miller, P. and Hyde, G. (1993b) 'Ways of coping with chronic fatigue syndrome: development of an illness management questionnaire', *Social Science and Medicine* 37(3), 385–91.

Richards, M. (1991) Letter, *Meeting Place* 36, 51–2.

Rodgers, S. (1992) 'Tired or toxic?', *Meeting-Place* 37, 26–8.

Roht, L. H., Vernon, S. W., Weir, F. W., Pier, S. M., Sullivan, P. and Reed, L. J. (1985) 'Community exposure to hazardous waste disposal sites: assessing reporting bias', *American Journal of Epidemiology* 122, 418–33.

Rosen, S. D., King, J. C., Wilkinson, J. B. and Nixon, P. G. (1990) 'Is chronic fatigue syndrome synonymous with effort syndrome?', *Journal of the Royal Society of Medicine* 83(12), 761–4.

Rowe, P. C., Bou-Holaigah, I., Kan, J. S. and Calkins, H. (1995) 'Is neurally mediated hypotension an unrecognised cause of chronic fatigue?', *Lancet* 345(8950), 623–4.

Russo, J., Katon, W., Sullivan, M., Clark, M. and Buchwald, D. (1994) 'Severity of somatization and its relationship to psychiatric disorders and personality', *Psychosomatics* 35, 546–56.

Saisch, S. G., Deale, A., Gardner, W. N. and Wessely, S. (1994) 'Hyperventilation and chronic fatigue syndrome', *Quarterly Journal of Medicine* 87(1), 63–7.

Salovey, P., O'Leary, A., Stretton, M. S., Fishkin, S. A. and Drake, C. A. (1991) 'Influence of mood on judgements about health and illness', in J. P. Firgas (ed), *Emotion and social judgements*, New York: Pergamon Press.

Scheffers, M. K., Johnson, S. K., Grafman, J., Dale, J. K. and Straus, S. E. (1992) 'Attention and short-term memory in chronic fatigue syndrome patients: an event-related potential analysis', *Neurology* 42, 1667–75.

Schluederberg, A., Straus, S. E., Peterson, P., Blumenthal, S., Komaroff, A. L., Spring, S. B., Landay, A. and Buchwald, D. (1992) NIH conference. 'Chronic fatigue syndrome research. Definition and medical outcome assessment', *Annals of Internal Medicine* 117(4), 325–31.

Schmaling, K. B. and DiClementi, J. D. (1995) 'Interpersonal stressors in chronic fatigue syndrome: a pilot study', *Journal of Chronic Fatigue*

Syndrome 1, 153–8.

Schmaling, K. B. and Jones, J. F. (1996) 'MMPI profiles of patients with chronic fatigue syndrome', *Journal of Psychosomatic Research* 40, 67–74.

Schwartz, R. B., Garada, B. M., Komaroff, A. L., Tice, H. M., Gleit, M., Jolesz, F. A. and Holman, B. L. (1994a) 'Detection of intracranial abnormalities in patients with chronic fatigue syndrome: comparison of MR imaging and SPECT', *American Journal of Roentgenology* 162(4), 935–41.

Schwartz, R. B., Komaroff, A. L., Garada, B. M., Gleit, M., Doolittle, T. H., Bates, D. W., Vasile, R. G. and Holman, B. L. (1994b) 'SPECT imaging of the brain: comparison of findings in patients with chronic fatigue syndrome, AIDS dementia complex, and major unipolar depression', *American Journal of Roentgenology* 162(4), 943–51.

Schweitzer, R., Kelly, B., Foran, A., Terry, D. and Whiting, J. (1995) 'Quality of life in chronic fatigue syndrome', *Social Science and Medicine* 41, 1367–72.

Scott, L. V. and Dinan, T. G. (1998) 'Urinary free cortisol excretion in chronic fatigue syndrome, major depression and in healthy volunteers', *Journal of Affective Disorders* 47(1–3), 49–54.

Scott, L. V., Medbak, S. and Dinan, T. G. (1998) 'Blunted adrenocorticotropin and cortisol responses to corticotropin-releasing hormone stimulation in chronic fatigue syndrome', *Acta Psychiatrica Scandinavica* 97, 450–547.

Shafran, S. D. (1991) 'The chronic fatigue syndrome', *American Journal of Medicine* 90, 730–9.

Sharpe, M., Clements, A., Hawton, K., Young, A. H., Sargent, P. and Cowen, P. J. (1996a) 'Increased prolactin response to buspirone in chronic fatigue syndrome', *Journal of Affective Disorders* 41(1), 71–6.

Sharpe, M., Hawton, K., Seagroatt, V. and Pasvol, G. (1992) 'Follow up of patients presenting with fatigue to an infectious diseases clinic', *British Medical Journal* 305, 147–52.

Sharpe, M., Hawton, K., Simkin, S., Surawy, C., Hackmann, A., Klimes, I., Peto, T., Warrell, D. and Seagroatt, V. (1996b) 'Cognitive behaviour therapy for the chronic fatigue syndrome: a randomized controlled trial', *British Medical Journal* 312(7022), 22–6.

Sharpe, M. C., Archard, L. C., Bantavala, J. E., Borysiewicz, L. K., Clare, A. W., David, A., Edwards, R. H. T., Hawton, K. E. H., Lambert, H. P., Lane, R. J. M., McDonald, E. M., Mowbray, J. F., Pearson, D. J., Peto, T. E. A., Preedy, V. R., Smith, A. P., Smith, D. G., Taylor, D. J., Tyrell, D. A., Wessely, S. and White, P. D. (1991) 'A report – chronic fatigue syndrome: guidelines for research', *Journal of the Royal Society of Medicine* 84, 118–21.

Shefer, A., Dobbins, J. G., Fukuda, K., Steele, L., Koo, D., Nisenbaum, R.

and Rutherford, G. W. (1997) 'Fatiguing illness among employees in three large state office buildings, California 1993 – was there an outbreak?', *Journal of Psychiatric Research* 31(1), 31–43.

Shorter, E. (1992) *From Paralysis to Fatigue: A History of Psychosomatic Illness in the Modern Era*, New York: The Free Press.

Shorter, E. (1993) 'Chronic fatigue in historical perspective', Ciba Foundation Symposium 173, 6–16; discussion 16–22.

Shorter, E. (1994) *From the Mind into the Body: The Cultural Origins of Psychosomatic Symptoms*, New York: The Free Press.

Shorter, E. (1995) 'Sucker-punched again: physicians meet the disease-of-the-month syndrome' (editorial), *Journal of Psychosomatic Research* 39(2), 115–8.

Simon, G. E., Katon, W. J. and Sparks, P. J. (1990) 'Allergic to life: psychological factors in environmental illness', *American Journal of Psychiatry* 147, 901–6.

Sisto, S. A., LaManca, J., Cordero, D. L., Bergen, M. T., Ellis, S. P., Drastal, S., Boda, W. L., Tapp, W. N. and Natelson, B. H. (1996) 'Metabolic and cardiovascular effects of a progressive exercise test in patients with chronic fatigue syndrome', *American Journal of Medicine* 100(6), 634–40.

Sisto, S. A., Tapp, W. N., Lamanca, J. J., Ling, W., Korn, L. R., Nelson, A. J. and Natelson, B. H. (1998) 'Physical activity before and after exercise in women with chronic fatigue syndrome', *Monthly Journal of the Association of Physicians* 91(7), 465–73.

Skelton, J. A. and Pennebaker, J. W. (1982) 'The psychology of physical symptoms and sensations', in G. S. Sanders and J. Suls (eds), *Social Psychology of Health and Illness*, Hillsdale, NJ: Erlbaum.

Smith, T. W., Follick, M. J., Ahern, D. K. and Adams, A. (1986) 'Cognitive distortion and disability in chronic low back pain', *Cognitive Therapy and Research* 10, 201–10.

Smith, T. W., Peck, J. R., Milano, R. A. and Ward, J. R. (1988) 'Cognitive distortion in rheumatoid arthritis: relation to depression and disability', *Journal of Consulting and Clinical Psychology* 56, 412–6.

Steinberg, P., McNutt, B. E., Marshall, P., Schenck, C., Lurie, N., Pheley, A. and Peterson, P. K. (1996) 'Double-blind placebo-controlled study of the efficacy of oral terfenadine in the treatment of chronic fatigue syndrome', *Journal of Allergy and Clinical Immunology* 97(1 Pt 1), 119–26.

Steincamp, J. (1989) *Overload: Beating M.E. The Chronic Fatigue Syndrome*, London: Fontana.

Stores, G., Fry, A. and Crawford, C. (1998) 'Sleep abnormalities demonstrated by home polysomnography in teenagers with chronic fatigue syndrome', *Journal of Psychosomatic Research* 45(1), 85–91.

Straus, S. E., Dale, J. K., Tobi, M., Lawley, T., Preble, O., Blaese, R. M., Hallahan, C. and Henle, W. (1988a) 'Acyclovir treatment of the chronic fatigue syndrome. Lack of efficacy in a placebo-controlled trial', *New England Journal of Medicine* 319(26), 1692–8.

Straus, S. E., Dale, J. K., Wright, R. and Metcalfe, D. D. (1988b) 'Allergy and the chronic fatigue syndrome', *Journal of Allergy and Clinical Immunology* 81(5 Pt 1), 791–5.

Straus, S. E., Fritz, S., Dale, J. K., Gould, B. and Strober, W. (1993) 'Lymphocyte phenotype and function in the chronic fatigue syndrome', *Journal of Clinical Immunology* 13(1), 30–40.

Straus, S. E., Tosato, G., Armstrong, G., Lawley, T., Preble, O. T., Henle, W., Davey, R., Pearson, G., Epstein, J., Brus, I. *et al.* (1985) 'Persisting illness and fatigue in adults with evidence of Epstein–Barr virus infection', *Annals of Internal Medicine* 102(1), 7–16.

Strickland, P., Morriss, R., Wearden, A. and Deakin, B. (1998) 'A comparison of salivary cortisol in chronic fatigue syndrome, community depression and healthy controls', *Journal of Affective Disorders* 47(1–3) 191–4.

Struewing, J. P. and Gray, G. C. (1990) 'An epidemic of respiratory complaints excaerbated by mass psychogenic illness in a military recruit population', *American Journal of Epidemiology* 132, 1120–9.

Sullivan, R. L. (1995) 'Chronic fee syndrome', *Forbes* 155, 114.

Surawy, C., Hackmann, A., Hawton, K. and Sharpe, M. (1995) 'Chronic fatigue syndrome: a cognitive approach', *Behaviour Research and Therapy* 33(5), 535–44.

Swanink, C. M. A., Vercoulen, J. H. M. M., Bleijenberg, G., Fennis, J. F. M., Galama, J. M. D. and van der Meer, J. W. M. (1995) 'Chronic fatigue syndrome: a clinical and laboratory study with a well matched control group', *Journal of Internal Medicine* 237, 499–506.

Thompson, D. (1992) 'Immune Dis-ease', *Mental Health News* Summer, 26–28.

Tirelli, U., Marotta, G., Improta, S. and Pinto, A. (1994) 'Immunological abnormalities in patients with chronic fatigue syndrome', *Scandinavian Journal of Immunology* 40, 601–8.

Turnquist, D. C., Harvey, J. H. and Andersen, B. L. (1988) 'Attributions and adjustment to life threatening illness', *British Journal of Clinical Psychology* 27, 17–22.

Unwin, C., Blatchley, N., Coker, W., Ferry, S., Hotopf, M., Hull, L., Ismail, K., Palmer, I., David, A. and Wessely, S. (1999) 'Health of UK servicemen who served in Persian Gulf War', *Lancet* 353(9148), 169–78.

Van Houdenhove, B., Onghena, P., Neerinckx, E. and Hellin, J. (1995) 'Does high 'action-proneness' make people more vulnerable to chronic fatigue syndrome? A controlled psychometric study', *Journal of Psychosomatic Research* 39, 633–640.

Vercoulen, J., Bazelmans, E., Swanink, C. M. A., Fennis, J. F. M., Galama, J. M. D., Jongen, P. J. H., Hommes, O., Vandermeer, J. W. M. and Bleijenberg, G. (1997) 'Physical activity in chronic fatigue syndrome –

assessment and its role in fatigue', *Journal of Psychiatric Research* 31(6), 661–73.

Vercoulen, J., Swanink, C. M. A., Zitman, F. G., Vreden, S. G. S., Hoofs, M. P. E., Fennis, J. F. M., Galama, J. M. D., Vandermeer, J. W. M. and Bleijenberg, G. (1996a) 'Randomised, double-blind, placebo-controlled study of fluoxetine in chronic fatigue syndrome', *Lancet* 347(9005), 858–61.

Vercoulen, J. H. M. M., Swanink, C. M. A., Fennis, J. F. M., Galama, J. M. D., van der Meer, J. W. M. and Bleijenberg, G. (1996b) 'Prognosis in chronic fatigue syndrome; a prospective study on the natural course', *Journal of Neurology, Neurosurgery and Psychiatry* 60, 489–94.

Vercoulen, J. H. M. M., Swanink, C. M. A., Fennis, J. F. M., Galama, J. M. D., van der Meer, J. W. M. and Bleijenberg, G. (1994) 'Dimensional assessment of chronic fatigue syndrome', *Journal of Psychosomatic Research* 38, 383–92.

Vollmer-Conna, U., Hickie, I., Hadzi-Pavlovic, D., Tymms, K., Wakefield, D., Dwyer, J. and Lloyd, A. (1997) 'Intravenous immunoglobulin is ineffective in the treatment of patients with chronic fatigue syndrome', *American Journal of Medicine* 103(1), 38–43.

Vollmer-Conna, U., Lloyd, A., Hickie, I. and Wakefield, D. (1998) 'Chronic fatigue syndrome: an immunological perspective', *Australian and New Zealand Journal of Psychiatry* 32(4), 523–7.

Ware, N. C. (1992) 'Suffering and the social construction of illness: the delegitimation of illness experience in chronic fatigue syndrome', *Medical Anthropology Quarterly* 6, 347–61.

Ware, N. C. (1993) 'Society, mind and body in chronic fatigue syndrome: an anthropological view', *Ciba Foundation Symposium* 173, 62–73; discussion 73–82.

Ware, N. C. (1998) 'Sociosomatics and illness in chronic fatigue syndrome', *Psychosomatic Medicine* 60(4), 394–401.

Ware, N. C. and Kleinman, A. (1992) 'Culture and somatic experience: the social course of illness in neurasthenia and chronic fatigue syndrome', *Psychosomatic Medicine* 54(5), 546–60.

Watson, D. and Pennebaker, J. W. (1989) 'Health complaints, stress, and distress: exploring the central role of negative affectivity', *Psycholological Review* 96(2), 234–54.

Wearden, A. J. and Appleby, L. (1996) 'Research on cognitive complaints and cognitive functioning in patients with chronic fatigue syndrome (CFS): what conclusions can we draw?', *Journal of Psychosomatic Medicine* 41, 197–211.

Wearden, A. J., Morriss, R. K., Mullis, R., Strickland, P. L., Pearson, D. J., Appleby, L., Campbell, I. T. and Morris, J. A. (1998) 'Randomised, double-blind, placebo-controlled treatment trial of fluoxetine and graded exercise for chronic fatigue syndrome', *British Journal of Psychiatry* 172,

485–90.

Weinman, J., Petrie, K. J., Moss-Morris, R. and Horne, R. (1996) 'The Illness Perception Questionnaire – a new method for assessing the cognitive representation of illness', *Psychology and Health* 11(3), 431–45.

Weinman, J., Petrie, K. J., Sharpe, N. and Walker, S. (in press) 'Causal attributions in patients and spouses following a heart attack and subsequent lifestyle changes', *British Journal of Health Psychology*.

Wessely, S. (1990) 'Old wine in new bottles: neurasthenia and ME', *Psychological Medicine* 20(1), 35–53.

Wessely, S. (1995a) 'Social and cultural aspects of chronic fatigue syndrome', *Journal of Musculoskeletal Pain* 3, 111–22.

Wessely, S. (1995c) 'Is neurally mediated hypotension an unrecognized cause of fatigue?' (letter to the editor), *Lancet* 345, 1112.

Wessely, S. (1996b) 'Chronic fatigue syndrome. Summary of a report of a joint committee of the Royal Colleges of Physicians, Psychiatrists and General Practitioners', *Journal of the Royal College of Physicians of London* 30(6), 497–504.

Wessely, S. (1997) 'Chronic fatigue syndrome: a 20th century illness?', *Scandinavian Journal of Work, Environment and Health* 23(Suppl. 3), 17–34.

Wessely, S. (1998) 'The epidemiology of chronic fatigue syndrome' (editorial), *Epidemiologia E Psichiatria Sociale* 7(1), 10–24.

Wessely, S., Butler, S., Chalder, T. and David, A. (1991) 'The cognitive behavioural management of the post-viral fatigue syndrome', in J. R. and J. Mowbrey (eds), *Postviral Fatigue Syndrome*, Chichester: John Wiley and Sons.

Wessely, S., Chalder, T., Hirsch, S., Pawlikowska, T., Wallace, P. and Wright, D. J. (1995b) 'Postinfectious fatigue: prospective cohort study in primary care', *Lancet* 345(8961), 1333–8.

Wessely, S., Chalder, T., Hirsch, S., Wallace, P. and Wright, D. (1996a) 'Psychological symptoms, somatic symptoms, and psychiatric disorder in chronic fatigue and chronic fatigue syndrome: a prospective study in the primary care setting', *American Journal of Psychiatry* 153(8), 1050–9.

Wessely, S., Chalder, T., Hirsch, S., Wallace, P. and Wright, D. (1997) 'The prevalence and morbidity of chronic fatigue and chronic fatigue syndrome: a prospective primary care study', *American Journal of Public Health* 87(9), 1449–55.

Wessely, S., Hotopf, M. and Sharpe, M. (1998) 'Treatment of CFS: the evidence', in *Chronic Fatigue and Its Syndromes*, Oxford: Oxford University Press.

Wessely, S., Nimnuan, C. and Sharpe, M. (1999) 'Functional somatic syndromes: one or many?', *Lancet* 354, 936–9.

Wessely, S. and Powell, R. (1989) 'Fatigue syndromes: a comparison of chronic 'postviral' fatigue with neuromuscular function', *Journal of Neurology, Neurosurgery and Psychiatry* 52, 940–8.

Whelton, C. L., Salit, I. and Moldofsky, H. (1992) 'Sleep, Epstein–Barr virus infection, musculoskeletal pain, and depressive symptoms in chronic fatigue syndrome', *Journal of Rheumatology* 19(6), 939–43.

White, P. (1989) 'Fatigue syndrome: neurasthenia revived', *British Medical Journal* 298, 1199–1200.

White, P. D., Thomas, J. M., Amess, J., Grover, S. A., Kangro, H. O. and Clare, A. W. (1995) 'The existence of a fatigue syndrome after glandular fever', *Psychological Medicine* 25(5), 907–16.

Williams, G., Pirohamed, J., Minors, D., Waterhouse, J., Buchan, I., Arendt, J. and Edwards, R. H. T. (1996) 'Dissociation of body-temperature and melatonin secretion circadian rhythms in patients with chronic fatigue syndrome', *Clinical Physiology* 16, 327–37.

Wilson, A., Hickie, I., Lloyd, A., Hadzi-Pavlovic, D., Boughton, C., Dwyer, J. and Wakefield, D. (1994a) 'Longitudinal study of outcome of chronic fatigue syndrome', *British Medical Journal* 308(6931), 756–9.

Wilson, A., Hickie, I., Lloyd, A., Hadzi-Pavlovic, D. and Wakefield, D. (1995) 'Cell-mediated immune function and the outcome of chronic fatigue syndrome', *International Journal of Immunopharmacology* 17(8), 691–4.

Wilson, A., Hickie, I., Lloyd, A. and Wakefield, D. (1994b) 'The treatment of chronic fatigue syndrome: science and speculation', *American Journal of Medicine* 96(6), 544–50.

Wood, B., Wessely, S., Papadopoulos, A., Poon, L., Checkley, S. (1998) 'Salivary cortisol profiles in chronic fatigue syndrome', *Neuropsychology* 37(1), 1–4.

Wood, G. C., Bentall, R. P., Göpfert, M. and Edwards, R. H. T. (1991) 'A comparative psychiatric assessment of patients with chronic fatigue syndrome and muscle disease', *Psychological Medicine* 21, 619–28.

Wood, P. (1941) 'Aetiology of Da Costa's syndrome', *British Medical Journal* 1, 845–51.

Wookey, C. (1986) *Myalgic Encephalomyelitis. Post-viral Fatigue Syndrome and How to Cope with it*, London: Croom Helm.

Yatham, L. N., Morehouse, R. L., Chisholm, B. T., Haase, D. A., MacDonald, D. D. and Marrie, T. J. (1995) 'Neuroendocrine assessment of serotonin (5-HT) function in chronic fatigue syndrome', *Canadian Journal of Psychiatry – Revue Canadienne de Psychiatrie* 40(2), 93–6.

Young, A. H., Sharpe, M., Clements, A., Dowling, B., Hawton, K. E. and Cowen, P. J. (1998) 'Basal activity of the hypothalamic–pituitary–adrenal axis in patients with the chronic fatigue syndrome (neurasthenia)', *Biological Psychiatry* 43(3), 236–7.

Zubieta, J. K., Demitrack, M. A., Shipley, J. E., Engleberg, N. C., Eiser, A. and Douglas, A. (1993) 'Sleep EEG in chronic fatigue syndrome:

comparison with major depression', paper presented at the Annual Meeting of the Society for Biological Psychiatry, San Francisco.

Zubieta, J. K., Engleberg, N. C., Yargic, L. I., Pande, A. C. and Demitrack, M. A. (1994) 'Seasonal symptoms variation in patients with chronic fatigue: comparison with major mood disorders', *Journal of Psychiatric Research* 28, 13–22.

Index